Covert Genocide

The Plot to Use Birth Control, Abortion, Sterilizations, and Gun Control to Exterminate the Black Race

By Anonymous

ISBN-13: 978-0615682211
ISBN-10: 0615682219

Table of Contents

Introduction

Conspiracy theorist! The phrase conjures up images of a strange, paranoid weirdo. We are told by the media that conspiracies about the rich and powerful are nonsense. But do conspiracies exist? The fact is that we are surrounded by conspiracies. The history of the world is a story of conspiracies. Are you a conspiracy theorist? Do you believe that a group of senators led by Brutus formed a conspiracy to kill Julius Caesar? Yes, how come this doesn't make you a conspiracy theorist? In fact, if you said that the idea that Brutus formed a conspiracy with a group of senators to kill Julius Caesar is just conspiracy theory and it never happened, people would look at you as a nut.

The newspapers are filled with conspiracies. Some of them are stranger than fiction. What if I told you that there is an international conspiracy of politicians and rabbis involved in graft and the trafficking of human organs and fake Gucci handbags? Am I conspiracy theorist? Not according to the FBI.

On July 23, 2009, the FBI arrested forty-four people in connection with this conspiracy. What if I told you that the existence of a secret society of Italian-Americans, named the Mafia, that is engaged in organized crime is just conspiracy theory and that there is no Mafia, and that anyone who believes the Mafia exists is a wacko conspiracy theorist? You would laugh at me, and you would be right to do so. Everyone knows the Mafia exists. But, did you know that at the height of Mafia's power, the official position of J. Edgar Hoover, the head of the FBI, and others in law enforcement was that the Mafia did not exist and that those who believed in the existence of the Mafia were conspiracy theorists? As the Mafia has lost power, the more its existence has become common knowledge. This is one of the important laws of conspiracies:

The more powerful the conspiracy the more able it is to hide its existence and dismiss those who expose them as conspiracy theorists.

When the Mafia was at height of its power, even the director of the FBI denied their existence. Now the Mafia is weak and movies and television shows are made about it.

In this book I will present evidence of a conspiracy far more powerful and insidious than the Mafia. The goal of these conspirators is not to acquire wealth but to eliminate up to 80 percent of the human race. Even more surprising than this shocking allegation is that the perpetrators have been open about their methods and goals. Some of the world's richest families, most respected foundations, and most powerful politicians are behind this campaign of genocide. They are motivated by a school of thought called eugenics.

Eugenics is a theory derived from Charles Darwin's theory of evolution which states that species change over time. This evolution results from what Darwin called "natural selection." Natural selection is the process in which superior members of a species outlive and outbreed less superior members. In short, Darwin believed that there is a "struggle for existence," and those individual members of a species that have traits to survive the struggle will have more offspring than members of the species that don't possess those traits. Eventually, through generations of natural selection, a new species will emerge. Eugenicists believe that, through evolution, the human race can evolve into a new superior species, a god-like super race. This super race will create a heaven on earth. There will be no crime and no wars and the super race will be immortal. But there is a catch. This evolutionary process cannot happen naturally. They believe that because of the advancement of technology and the economic progress created by free markets, natural selection no longer eliminates the weakest members of our species. These weak members, whom they often call "human waste," are preventing the super race from evolving. The eugenicists believe if the "human waste" cannot be eliminated naturally; they must be eliminated unnaturally. Just exactly who is "human waste"? Most eugenicists believe that at least 80 percent of the human race is "human waste." In some races the figure is even higher. They believe, for instance, that 100 percent of the black race is human waste. Therefore, all blacks must be eliminated.

How do you eliminate 80 percent of the people on planet earth? How do you kill all black people on the planet? This is the most pressing question for the eugenicists. During the beginning of the twentieth century, some advocated "fast kill" solutions, while others preferred a more patient, long-term "slow kill" approach. Adolph Hitler, an avid eugenicist, preferred the "fast kill" approach. He, as we know, used lethal gas chambers to eliminate those he deemed to be "human waste." Despite the thousands of people he killed, Hitler is considered a failure by modern eugenicists. Not only did he not eliminate all human waste, but he also caused eugenics to receive a tremendous amount of negative publicity. Today, the consensus among eugenicists is to use a "slow kill" approach. These tactics include contaminated vaccinations, the promotion of birth control, abortion, and sterilizations. This book will outline how the modern eugenicists are using these tactics in their quest to eliminate the black race.

Chapter 1: The Origins

Sir Francis Galton, an Englishman and cousin of Charles Darwin, coined the term eugenics and first popularized its theories. Galton, drawing heavily on his cousin's theory of evolution and the process of natural selection, postulated that if humans' reproduction activities could be controlled, improvements could be made to the human race. He believed that if people were bred just as we breed pigs or horses, then this would allow "more suitable races or strains of blood a better chance of prevailing over the less suitable"[1] Galton defined Eugenics as "the science of improvement of the human race germ plasm through better breeding."[2]

Galton advocated selective breeding for humans in order to create a super race. He declared that his research made it "quite practicable to produce a highly gifted race of men by

---

1 Phillip D. Collins, "Engineering Evolution: The Alchemy of Eugenics," http://www.conspiracyarchive.com/Commentary/Evolution.htm, 10 January 2005.
2 Ibid.

judicious marriages during several consecutive generations" and eventually this would create a god-like class of "prophets and high priests of civilization into the world."[3]

Galton felt nothing but contempt for the average man:

"The average man is morally and intellectually an uninteresting being . . . of no direct help towards evolution."[4]

For Galton, man's only purpose was to advance evolution. Galton, of course, disagreed with the Christian view that all men are created equally in the image of God. In Galton's worldview there were two types of people: those who could advance the evolutionary process and those who would hinder or reverse the evolutionary process, a process called dysgenics. His fear of dysgenics led him not only to hold most of humanity in contempt but also to view the procreation of the inferior classes of people as a grave threat to the world. Galton wrote, "If the poorer stock continued to procreate children, 'inferior' in

---

3 William H. Tucker, *The Science of Politics and Racial Research*
University of Illinois Press, 1994, 46.
4 Ibid. 45.

moral, intellectual and physical qualities, the time come when such persons would be considered as enemies to the state, and to have forfeited all claims to kindness."[5]

Blacks were one of the races he believed to be of "poorer stock" or a "low race" and therefore a future threat to the civilized world. Although he did believe that there were a few blacks of "good stock," the overwhelming majority were of "poor stock." Because so many blacks were of "poor stock," selective breeding of blacks would not be feasible as it would be with whites. Therefore, to advance the evolutionary process, the black race must be eliminated. He proposed eliminating blacks by having them displaced with a superior race, the Chinese. Chinese people would be relocated to Africa, and a Darwinian "survival of the fittest" struggle would ensue. The Chinese would win this struggle, and the blacks would be displaced and they would eventually become an extinct race. Galton wrote, "The gain would be immense to the whole civilized world if he were to outbreed and finally displace the Negro."[6]

---

5 Ibid. 48.
6 Ibid., 49.

To the modern ear Galton sounds like some sort of kook who we would find on the Jerry Springer show. He certainly does not sound like a distinguished professor, roaming the halls of universities, giving lectures to academia. Galton was not an ostracized member of the lunatic fringe; he was a well-respected member of the scientific community, with a significant following. The science he created, eugenics, would be studied and taught at the most prestigious institutions and received generous funding from wealthy philanthropists. The list of institutions and families that gave financial support and promoted eugenics reads like a Who's Who of American establishment: the Carnegie Institution, the Rockefeller Foundation, the Harriman family, Harvard University, Princeton University, Yale University, Stanford University, the American Medical Association, Supreme Court Justice Oliver Wendell Holmes, Woodrow Wilson, the American Museum of Natural History, and the State Department are just some of organizations and people behind the eugenics movement.[7]

---

[7] Edwin Black, *War Against the Weak: Eugenics and America's Campaign to Create a Master Race* : Four Walls Eight Windows, 2003, XXI–XXII.

The Carnegie foundation was one of the first to fund the eugenics movement when it gave a grant to Charles Davenport to establish the Biological Experiment Station at Cold Spring Harbor to study and promote eugenics in 1902.[8] In 1911 the Carnegie Foundation funded a study that issued a report called the "Preliminary Report of the Committee of the Eugenic Section of the American Breeder's Association to Study and to Report on the Best Practical Means for Cutting Off the Defective Germ-Plasm in the Human Population." "Defective Germ-Plasm" is the eugenicists' phrase for people they deem inferior and want to eliminate. The report praised the Spartan practice of drowning weak children, because they would be of no use to society. It had eighteen suggestions to stop "defectives" from having children; the eighth solution openly called for genocide.[9]

Nobel Peace Prize winner and socialist George Bernard Shaw also called for the killing of undesirables and stated, "A part of eugenics politics would finally land us in an extensive

---

[8] Ibid., 36.
[9] Ibid., 247.

use of the lethal chamber. A great many people would have to be put out of existence, simply because it wastes other people's time to look after them."[10]

Despite having support from some of the most influential people in America, the eugenicists faced substantial obstacles. How were they to carry out their theories? Attempts to limit the birthrate of any segment of the population would certainly result in resistance from the target groups and from other organizations, like churches. In their perfect world they could round up all those deemed "unfit" and execute them in gas chambers, but fortunately the American public would not tolerate such a practice. Any eugenics program must be kept secret. It could not survive in the light. The eugenicists understood the difficulties they faced. So, they moved slowly under various pretexts, careful not to reveal their true intentions. Like guerrilla warriors fighting an enemy with more troops, better technology, and more resources, they prepared for a long war and did not mind losing the occasional battle. Guerrilla

---

[10] Ibid., 248.

fighters know if they face a conventional army head on, their full force against the enemy's full force, they will lose. As Chinese Communist leader Mao Zedong concisely summed up the strategy of counterinsurgents, "The enemy advances, we retreat. The enemy camps, we harass. The enemy tires, we attack. The enemy retreats, we pursue." Guerilla war is a war of attrition. The eugenicists are following Mao's advice and are fighting a long multigenerational war of attrition. This war is fought on mostly two fronts: the political front and the public opinion front. On the political front the eugenicists must get governments to enact eugenic legislation. On the public opinion front they must change public opinion to ensure there will be no grassroots opposition to their plans.

On both fronts the eugenicists must move slowly. They can't just go round up millions of people and put them in gas chambers, because this would provoke a wide-scale backlash from the American people, a backlash so great that they would never be able to recover. Their plans would be exposed and the public would always be on watch for anyone promoting any form of eugenics legislation. Any attempt to enact a eugenics program would be immediately shot down. The eugenicists use a similar strategy commonly used to boil a frog. If you throw a frog into a pot of boiling water, it will just jump out of the pot, but if you put the frog into a pot of cool water and slowly raise the temperature, the frog will never realize it is being boiled alive and won't leave the pot.

Chapter 2: Hitler and Eugenics

In Germany, there was one man who was deeply influenced by the eugenicist movement. That man's name was Adolph Hitler. While Hitler was serving time in prison in the 1920s, he poured over the works and textbooks of American eugenicists. He even sent fan mail to Leon Whitney, president of the American Eugenics Society (AES), and eugenics writer Madison Grant, the author of *The Passing of the Great Race*. Hitler was particularly fond of *The Passing of the Great Race*, which he called his "bible." [11] A look inside Hitler's bible shows that it completely rejects the tenets of Christianity and the belief in moral absolutes. Grant wrote, "Mistaken regard for what are believed to be divine laws and a sentimental belief in the sanctity of human life tend to prevent both the elimination of defective infants and the sterilization of such adults as are themselves of no value to the community. The laws of nature require the obliteration of the unfit and human life is valuable only when it is of use to the community or race"[12]

The Passing of the Great Race was a best seller and received many favorable reviews.[13] In this book Hitler found his racist belief that the Aryans, or Nordics, were the superior race destined to rule mankind and that all other races, including the Jews, were inferior. Grant's ideas were also influential on his friend, Congressman Albert Johnson, chairman of Congress's Immigration and Naturalization Committee.[14] Based on the committee's recommendations, Congress passed laws

---

[11] Ibid., 259.
[12] Ibid.
[13] Tucker, *The Science of Politics and Racial Research,* 2.
[14] Black, *War against the Weak,* 192.

establishing racial quotas that gave preference to northern Europeans.

When Hitler became chancellor in 1933, he, unlike his American counterparts, had no constraints on his power, and he was free to initiate eugenic policies without any fear of public backlash or resistance. He started a positive eugenics program, the encouragement of the birth of desirable peoples, and a negative eugenics program, the discouragement or outright prevention of the birth of undesirable peoples. As part of his positive eugenics program, gold medals were given to Aryan women with eight or more children. Interest free loans were awarded to newlyweds with one-fourth of the loan forgiven for each child that was born. Propaganda films and lectures encouraged women to have birth.[15] These were just some of the incentives given to increase the birthrate of racially superior Germans.

Hitler borrowed methods from the Americans in his campaign to eliminate the bad gene pool, and he developed his

---

[15] Robert G. Weisbord, *Genocide?: Birth Control and the Black American.* Greenwood Press, 1975, 58–60.

own tactics that American eugenicists would eventually adopt and implement. He promoted birth control, abortion, pornography, homosexuality, sterilization, and basic general moral degradation among the classes he wanted to eliminate. Below is a summary of his tactics:

1.) **Birth control** - Contraceptives were outlawed for Aryans but made legal for the "inferior" races and those living in the occupied territories. Hitler explained this dichotomy by saying, "Active trade in contraceptives ought to be actually encouraged in the Eastern territories, as we could not possibly have the slightest interest in increasing the non-German population."[16] Clever propaganda came along with the legalization of birth control to persuade people to use birth control and not have children. This was especially necessary in Catholic countries, because the Church taught and continues to teach its members that birth control is a mortal sin. Pro birth control propaganda reminded families how costly it is to have

---

[16] Elasah Drogin, *Margaret Sanger: Father of Modern Society*. CUL Publications, 1989, p. 24.

and raise children. They were also told that childbirth is extremely dangerous to a woman's health. A Nazi memorandum stated, "Every propaganda means, especially the press, radio, and movies, as well as pamphlets, booklets, and lectures, must be used to instill in the Russian population the idea that it is harmful to have several children. We must emphasize the expenses that children cause, the good things that people could have had with the money spent on them. We could also hint at the dangerous effect of child-bearing on a woman's health."[17]

2.)   **Abortion** – Like contraceptives, abortions was also outlawed for Aryans but legalized for those from bad gene pools. Speaking about the occupied Eastern territories, Hitler said, "In view of the large families of the native population, it could only suit us if the girls and women there had as many abortions as possible."[18] A memorandum issued from Berlin

---

[17] Mike W. Perry, "As Many Abortions as Possible," http://www.ewtn.com/library/PROLIFE/NAZIPOPU.TXT, 17 September 2009.
[18] Drogin, *Margaret Sanger*, 24.

declared, "It will even be necessary to open special institutions for abortion, and to train midwives and nurses for this purpose. The population will practice abortion all the more willingly if these institutions are competently operated. The doctors must be able to help out there being any question of this being a breach of their professional ethics."[19]

3.)   **Promotion of Homosexuality, Pornography, and the General Moral Degeneration -** Hitler outlawed homosexuality in Germany but legalized it in Poland. Homosexual sex is viewed as the ideal sexual relationship for the "unfit" because people can satisfy their natural sexual urges without any risk of anyone getting pregnant. Eugenicists know that people are always going to have sex. So the idea is not to get everyone to take a vow of celibacy, but rather to get people to have sex only for pleasure. They do not want people to view sex as a way to consummate a marriage and to have children. As promiscuity and sex outside of marriage becomes more acceptable fewer

---

[19] Perry, "As Many Abortions as Possible.".

people get married and fewer children are born. In order to get people to lose their traditional values about sex and marriage the Germans promoted and distributed pornography in the Eastern territories.

> The German Propaganda Office . . . was supposed to organize or sponsor Polish burlesque shows and publish cheap literature, strongly erotic in nature . . . to keep the masses on a low level and to divert their interest from political aspirations. These projects for degeneration and moral debasement were actually realized in the larger Polish cities. . . . German success in this effort was significant enough to become a target of the Polish Underground. The latter used to dispatch some special "punishing squads" which overran some of the ill-famed Variety Theaters and took disciplinary measures against the Polish collaborators in the programs.[20]

The overt attempt to destroy the moral fiber of the occupied territories also had military and strategic benefits. It would

---

[20] Ibid.

weaken any military resistance to the German occupation because immoral and nihilistic people have less will to fight than religious and principled peoples. Trying to destroy the morals of your enemies is not unique to the Germans. The Israelis borrowed this tactic from the Germans in April of 2002, when they took over Palestinian television stations and broadcasted pornography even during daytime hours when children were home.[21]

4.) **Sterilization** – Hitler passed sterilization laws that were almost verbatim of translated texts of American laws. One prominent eugenicist noted, "the text of the German statue reads almost like the 'American model sterilization law.'"[22] They even invented an X-ray machine to sterilize Jews that was the envy of Franklin D. Roosevelt, who told his advisers that he would like to use it on Puerto Ricans.[23] The Law for the Prevention of Progeny with Hereditary Diseases forcibly

---

[21] "Porn Run on Seized TV Channel, Say Residents," *Sunday Morning Herald*, 1 April 2002.
<http://www.smh.com.au/articles/2002/04/01/1017206174636.html>.
[22] Black, *War against the Weak*, 300.
[23] Perry, "As Many Abortions as Possible.".

23

sterilized those found "unfit." Between 320,000 and 350,000 people were sterilized under the Nazi regime.[24]

The Americans were watching the developments in Germany with mixture of envy and apprehension. Dictatorship brought Hitler certain advantages that a constitutional republic like the United States did not have. Hitler was free to enact any policy without worrying about public opinion or congressional objections. As George W. Bush once quipped about our form of government, "You don't get everything you want. A dictatorship would be a lot easier." Joseph DeJarnette, superintendent of Virginia's Western State Hospital, lamented that, "The Germans are beating us at our own game."[25]

The Germans and the Americans had a cooperative relationship. They held conferences and corresponded with each other, sharing ideas, successes, and failures. American eugenics journals began printing pro-Nazi articles that cited Nazis, including Dr. Otmar Freiherr von Vershuer, the man who

---

[24] Ibid.
[25] Black, *War against the Weak,* 277.

trained the notorious Dr. Joseph Mengele.[26] The Germans also praised the Americans, even awarding Dr. Harry Laughlin, director of the Harriman-funded Eugenics Record Office, with an honorary degree.[27] But American support of the Nazis was not limited to honorary degrees and verbal encouragement; they also provided financial support. The Rockefeller Foundation supplied over $125,000 for German eugenics research. Funding did not stop with the start of World War II. The Rockefeller Foundation funded experiments in concentration camps during WWII.[28]

Although American eugenicists mostly had praise for Hitler's negative eugenics plan (decreasing the birthrate of the "unfit"), they were critical of his positive eugenics program (increasing the birthrate of the superior Aryan race). The American eugenicists felt he should target the Aryan population and weed out the "unfit" among the Aryan race. In 1940 the general director of the Birth Control Federation of America,

---

[26] Ibid., 342–43.
[27] Ibid., 312.
[28] Ibid., 363–64.

Woodbridge Morris, told the Germans, "We, too, recognize the problem of race building, but our concern is with the quality of our people, not with their quantity alone." [29]

Despite some concerns, the American eugenicists were mostly excited about Hitler's eugenics program. They could learn from his mistakes and successes. But there were dangers. The world was watching Hitler. If Hitler went too far, exposed too much, and his ties to American eugenicists became public, the consequences could be disastrous. The term eugenics itself would never be able to recover from the awful smell of being connected with Hitler. No public relations campaign could wash away that smell, and it would it make it extremely difficult to carry out a far-reaching aggressive Nazi-like eugenics program in the United States. As one American eugenicist noted, "If Hitler succeeds in his wholesale sterilization, it will be a demonstration that will carry eugenics farther than a hundred Eugenics Societies could. If he makes a fiasco of it, it will set

---

[29] Perry, "As Many Abortions as Possible."

the movement back where a hundred eugenics societies can never resurrect it."[30]

Fortunately for mankind, Hitler did make a fiasco of it. Eugenics was universally condemned when the Nazis were defeated and the full extent of the Nazi eugenics program became public. The architects of the Nazi eugenics program were put on trial for their crimes at Nuremberg. The Nazi defeat and the resulting condemnation put the American elite in a quandary. They did not want to give up eugenics at home, and at the same time, if their links to the Nazi became too widely known it would be the death blow to eugenics. Giving up was not an option for the Americans. They decided to become more public relations savvy. They toned down their rhetoric. No longer would they make open and brutally frank public statements about eliminating "human weeds." They even changed the name. Eugenics would no longer be called eugenics; it would now be called "sustainable development," "family planning," "population control," "human engineering,"

---

[30] Black, *War against the Weak,* 317.

or "genetics."[31] Eugenics organizations took the eugenics out of their names. For instance, the American Eugenics Society became the Society for the Study of Social Biology and still exists today.[32] They became more guarded and less revealing. Today most Web sites of eugenic organizations restrict access to their site and only allow vetted users access.[33] But as we shall see, they did not stop their quest to create a master race.

Chapter 3: Margaret Sanger—Mother of Eugenics

In America, the eugenics movement has always been composed of two divisions: the think tanks that publish studies and propaganda to provide justification and the activist organizations that put the theories into practice. Margaret Sanger was the first general of the activist arm. No person has done more to advance eugenics in America than Sanger. She

---

[31] Ibid., 8.
[32] Ibid., 425.
[33] Ibid., XXIII.

helped find the most successful eugenics organization, the Birth Control League, now known as Planned Parenthood. She was instrumental in the development of the strategies and tactics that are still employed today by the eugenicists in their campaign to eliminate the "unfit" from the human race.

Margaret Sanger was born into a family of eleven children in Corning, New York, on September 14, 1879. Her father was an ardent anti-Christian who forbid his Catholic wife from giving their children a religious education. Despite her husband's orders, Margaret's mother secretly had Margaret baptized and confirmed. As a young girl, Margaret was a practicing Catholic despite her father's attempts to undermine her faith. Eventually, though, she grew to hate the Church.[34] Sanger grew up to be a beautiful, charming, and intelligent woman. After dropping out of high school, she married a wealthy architect named William Sanger and began a life as a housewife on New York's upper eastside. Margaret soon became bored with housework and began taking an interest in

---

[34] George Grant, *Killer Angel: A Short Biography of Planned Parenthood's Founder, Margaret Sanger* Highland Books, 2001 32.

communism, anarchism, and socialism. She met and was friends with the prominent radical anti-Christian thinkers of her day. Her circle of friends included feminist anarchist Emma Goldman; Havelock Ellis, a believer in sexual liberation; and socialist Eugene Debs. Margaret Sanger was most attracted to those ideologies that promoted promiscuous sex and eugenics. Her interest in free sex inspired her to ask her husband for an open marriage because she now felt marriage to be a "degenerate institution." Eventually, she and her husband divorced. After her divorce Margaret became more involved in radical politics and started to publish a pro-birth control newsletter. Birth control is the all-encompassing phrase for contraceptives (condoms), birth control pills, and sterilizations. Anything that allows people to have sex without out fear of the women getting pregnant would be considered birth control. In 1916 she founded the Birth Control League, later named Planned Parenthood. She was a gifted organizer, fund-raiser, and propagandist. Under Margaret's leadership, Planned Parenthood grew to be the premiere and most influential eugenics organization in the world. Margaret had found her passion in life. As of 2004 Planned Parenthood had $810 million in revenues annually, 850 clinics all over the world, and $725 million in assets.[35]

Early on Sanger was always honest about the goal of her organization; it was to create a master race and prevent the evolutionary degeneration of the human race. As Margaret Sanger phrased her goal, "More children from the fit, less from the unfit—is the chief aim of birth control."[36] Before Adolph Hitler gave eugenics a bad name Margaret Sanger's writings are remarkable for their brutal frankness. Later, like all eugenicists, she toned downed her rhetoric and even changed the name of her organization from the Birth Control League to the more innocuous sounding Planned Parenthood. Her early writings reveal her true thoughts and aims. One doesn't need to engage in any speculation to state that Sanger was a eugenicist launching a genocidal campaign against the human race because her own words speak for themselves and convict her.

---

[35] Planned Parenthood. *Annual Report, 2003–2004*
[36] Drogin, *Margaret Sanger,* 12.

Margaret Sanger's personal philosophy was marked by a hatred of the poor and the "human waste" and a belief that eventually through evolution a master race of "human thoroughbreds" [37,38] would emerge. Sanger's hatred of the poor was so extreme that she even despised charity because it "encourages the healthier and more normal sections of the world to shoulder the burden of unthinking and indiscriminate fecundity of others; which brings with it, as I think the reader must agree, a dead weight of *human waste*. Instead of decreasing and aiming to eliminate the stocks that are most detrimental to the future of the race and the world, it tends to render them to a menacing degree dominant."(emphasis mine).[39] In Sanger's stated opinion about 70 percent of the population was "feebleminded" and therefore a "menace to the race."[40]

In her book, *The Pivot of Civilization*, Sanger describes her utopian vision. In her ideal world, half the world's population would be segregated and sterilized. As Sanger puts

[37] Margaret Sanger, *The Pivot of Civilization*. Project Gutenberg, Web-E-book, 65.
[38] Ibid., 75
[39] Drogin, *Margaret Sanger,* 17.
[40] Ibid., 21.

it, "nearly one-half the entire population, will never develop mental capacity beyond the state of moron. . . . Our failure to segregate morons who are increasing and multiplying, though in truth I have merely scratched the surface of this international menace, demonstrates our foolhardy and extravagant sentimentalism."[41] Once the human waste was segregated from the rest of population, they would put to work as slave labor on farms, "where they would be taught to work under competent instructors for the period of their entire lives."[42] Eventually, the human waste would die out. Sanger called this her "Plan for Peace."[43]

After the "morons" were segregated from society, Sanger believed that a Utopian society that would emerge. She liked to call it a "terrestrial paradise."[44] Mankind would be free from "debauch of sentimentality or religiosity" and "by releasing their sexual energies . . . they could create a 'race of

---

[41] Ibid., 65.
[42] Phillip D. Collins, "Engineering Evolution: The Alchemy of Eugenics," http://www.conspiracyarchive.com/Commentary/Evolution.htm, 10 January 2005.
[43] Drogin, *Margaret Sanger,* 21.
[44] Ibid., 66.

geniuses.'"[45] By segregating those who are "biological and racial mistake . . . mankind may attain the great spiritual illumination which will transform the world, which will light up the only path to an earthly paradise."[46] Sanger was willing to sacrifice millions of innocent people in order to create this heaven on earth.

Eugenics cloaks itself as a science, but as can be seen from Sanger's description of heaven, it is actually a religion. Instead of believing in a God as a creator, they believe that man created himself. It is through eugenics that man can perfect his creation and create a race of Gods. Not all men are destined to be Gods; only the chosen ones. When you look at eugenics as a religion, you can understand their hatred for "human waste." The "human waste" is preventing them from becoming Gods.

The American establishment recognized Margaret Sanger's talents and viewed as her efforts as one of the best prospects to bring about a eugenics regime in America. The Rockefeller family, the Osborn family, and the Brush

---

[45] Ibid.
[46] Ibid.

foundation are just a few of her generous supporters. Albert

Einstein, Eleanor Roosevelt, H. G. Wells, Emperor Hirohito,

Dwight Eisenhower, Harry Truman, and Henry Ford are just

some of her admirers. In 2000 she was named one of *Time*

Magazine's one hundred most influential people in the

twentieth century, and she was even commemorated on a U.S.

postal stamp[47]. One of Sanger's most vocal admirers currently

is Hillary Clinton. Clinton had nothing but praises for Sanger's

life and works when accepting the Margaret Sanger Award from

Planned Parenthood in March of 2009, when she stated:

> I admire Margaret Sanger enormously, her courage, her
>
> tenacity, her vision . . . taking on archetypes, taking on
>
> attitudes and accusations flowing from all directions, I
>
> am really in awe of her. And there are a lot of lessons
>
> that we can learn from her life and from the cause she
>
> launched and fought for and sacrificed so bravely.
>
> The 20th century reproductive rights movement,
>
> really embodied in the life and leadership of Margaret

---

[47] Robert G. Weisbord, *Genocide?: Birth Control and the Black American*
Greenwood Press, 1975, 4.

Sanger, was one of the most transformational in the entire history of the human race. . . . Yet we know that Margaret Sanger's work here in the United States and certainly across our globe is not done.

Margaret Sanger was not a racist as the term is commonly understood today. She did not hate blacks, but just viewed them as inferior species. She also viewed most whites as inferior "human waste." Her racism was not based on the color of a person's skin; it was based on their genetics. In *The Pivot of Civilization*, she quotes a Dr. Freeman who explains that even some whites may be inferior to blacks: "Compared with the African negro, the British sub-man is in several respects markedly inferior. He tends to be dull; he is usually quite helpless and unhandy; he has, as a rule, no skill or knowledge of handicraft, or indeed knowledge of any kind"[48]

---

[48] Sanger, *The Pivot of Civilization,* 70.

Margaret Sanger viewed **most** whites as coming from a "defective gene pool" but she viewed **all** blacks as "human waste"

Unfortunately for Sanger, but fortunately for the rest of the world, Sanger couldn't just march blacks into gas chambers, like her buddy Hitler did to the Jews in Nazi German. To defend her eugenic utopian vision from the threat the black race posed, she devised a plan called the Negro Project.

Chapter 4: Negro Project

In internal memos the rational for the initiative was explained this way: "The mass of Negroes, particularly in the South, still breed carelessly and disastrously, with the result that the increase among Negroes, even more than among whites, is from that portion of the population least intelligent and fit, and least able to rear children properly."[49] Sanger's letters with colleagues, they openly show their disdain for blacks and state,

---

[49] Linda Gordon, *Woman's Body, Woman's Right : A Social History of Birth Control in America* Penguin Books, 1977, 332.

37

"Public health statistics merely hint at the primitive state of civilization in which most Negroes in the South live."[50] The goal was to eliminate the black race, but to accomplish such a diabolical goal without blacks catching on, Sanger would develop a cunning strategy and employ tactics of deception to hide their true intentions.

The Negro Project would use tactics identical to those used by Hitler against his enemies to lower the birth rate and gradually lead to the race's extinction:

1)   Promotion of birth control;

2)   Promotion of abortion;

3)   Forced and voluntary sterilizations;

4)   Promotion of moral degeneracy, including but not limited to promoting sex out wedlock and ending the shame of having bastard children.

At the time the Negro Project was devised, every one of the tactics listed above was considered an anathema by the

---

[50] Ibid., 332.

American people. Abortion was illegal. Contraceptive was illegal in many states, and the vast majority considered sex outside of marriage to be a sin. It was clear to Sanger and her cohorts that a public relations campaign would be needed to change peoples' opinions, particularly black peoples' opinions. Like a general who softens the enemy with a barrage of artillery and mortar fire before launching a ground offensive, Sanger launched a propaganda offensive to soften the ground before implementing her most aggressive tactics, like building abortion mills in black neighborhoods.

At first the principal targets of her propaganda were the black leaders of the community, particularly the secular black intelligentsia and black reverends. Sanger and her allies theorized that the best way and probably the only way to initiate a large-scale genocidal birth control campaign was to make it appear as if blacks were behind it. Their plan simply stated was, we can't kill them, so we must get them to kill themselves. Clarence Gamble, cofounder of Planned Parenthood, explained this strategy to future financial donor of the Negro Project,

Mary Lasker, wife of famous advertising executive Albert Lasker, this way: "There is great danger that we will fail because the Negroes think it a plan for extermination. Hence lets appear to let the colored ~~think it~~ run it [*sic*] as we appeared to let the south do the conference at Atlanta."[51] The strategy was by changing the minds of a small group of leaders in the black community, she could eventually change the minds of millions of blacks. These influential blacks could use their positions in academia, business, politics, or in the church to mold the opinions of the black masses on sexual moral issues and provide cover by serving as front men. As you will see, they were successful, and the black public's opinion on contraception, abortion, and the traditional two-parent family has dramatically changed. In essence, the goal of Sanger and her allies was to train and cultivate an army of black Judas goats. A Judas goat is used in slaughterhouses to lead sheep to their slaughter. The goat is trained to associate with the sheep and gain their trust. Once the sheep are comfortable with the

---

[51] Ibid., 333.

Judas goat, they will begin to follow the goat. One day the sheep will unwittingly follow the goat to the slaughterhouse to be killed. For his service, the Judas goat's life is spared.

The effort to promote birth control among blacks has to be understood in the context of the times. Now, most people consider not using contraceptives or not practicing so called "safe sex" as some sort of a secular "sin," but not too long ago most people considered the use of contraception as a sin against God and Nature. Even today, the largest church in America, the Roman Catholic Church, teaches that birth control of any sort to be a mortal sin. Before the widespread birth control propaganda of the eugenicists there was a consensus among Americans that sex should only be between married couples and birth control was immoral and ought to be outlawed. In fact, in 1873 Congress passed the Comstock Law, which prohibited the sale or promotion of contraceptives through the U.S. mail. Blacks, like whites, also viewed birth control as a sin, which was acknowledged by the only black founder member of the National Association for the Advancement of Colored People

(NAACP), W. E. B Du Bois, who wrote "they think that birth control is inherently immoral."[52]

It was obvious to Planned Parenthood that for their plan to work, black attitudes toward birth control must change. A study done in 1940 in Nashville, Tennessee, found that half of black mothers were against the use of contraception.[53] Nine years later the same study in Nashville found that only one-third of black mothers were against the use of birth control.[54] This remarkable change in attitudes can be attributed to the Negro Project's social engineering program to change black attitudes. This propaganda effort is continuing in the present day.

Planned Parenthood knew blacks would be suspicious if a bunch of white people who never had much to do with blacks, all of sudden, took a keen interest in blacks and went around telling them, "Stop having so many children. Use birth control. Get sterilized. Have abortions. It is for your own good." No, that wouldn't work. They needed black front men. A front man

---

[52] W. E. B. Du Bois, "Black Folk and Birth Control," *Birth Control Review* (June 1936): 166–67.
[53] Weisbord, *Genocide?*, 43.
[54] Ibid.

or organization looks to the public like it is serving one purpose but it in actuality serves a hidden ulterior purpose. The most commonly known fronts are front companies used by organized crime to launder money. Planned Parenthood recruited among black America's opinion molders (intellectuals, ministers, and politicians) to find front men.

They had their first great successes in getting front men from black America's intelligentsia. It is not surprising that intellectuals would find the elitist message of eugenics appealing. Remember, eugenicists do not discriminate by race, but by genetics. Because of their focus on genetics rather than on race, they have been called scientific racists. Just as it was possible for Margaret Sanger to despise most whites and want to see them exterminated, it is just as possible for a black person to despise most of his fellow blacks and want them eliminated. So it is not hard to understand how members of the black elite, particularly intellectuals who are naturally are aware of their intellectual superiority to the general population, could believe in eugenics. With black intellectuals Sanger was more honest and confided in them with her eugenic vision. They were told that were part of the genetically superior race of human beings and that majority of blacks as well as whites were "human waste" that needed to be eliminated. Black intellectuals were just as attracted to the ideas of eugenics as whites and became some of its most ardent supporters.

Planned Parenthood hit pay dirt in June 1932 when they were able to lure some of black America's leading intellectuals to their side. George S. Schuyler, a columnist and author; Charles S. Johnson, president of Fisk University; Elmer A. Carter, editor of the Urban League's journal *Opportunity*; and W. E. B. Du Bois, the first black man to get a Harvard PHD, all agreed to lend their names to Planned Parenthood's Negro Project. They all wrote pro-birth control articles in Planned Parenthood's flagship publication, at that time, the *Birth Control Review*. W. E. B. Du Bois was the prize catch, because as editor of the NAACP's flagship publication the *Crisis,* he was arguably black America's most famous and public figure at the time. Today, many schools are named after him and Harvard University founded the W. E. B. Du Bois Institute in his honor.

The *Birth Control Review* is an academic publication that would not be read by the masses or the working classes. It is clear from the articles that their goal is to convince the black intellectual classes that birth control should be promoted to the black underclass. The hope is that the intellectuals would write articles and give lectures on the usefulness and necessity of birth control. The idea would spread down from the intellectual class to the middle class to the lower class. This is one technique to change a target group's opinions and attitudes.

With articles entitled "Quantity or Quality" or "Eugenics for the Negro" these men did not hide their elitist attitudes and disdain for the majority of blacks in the pieces they wrote. By reading their words, one can gain insight into the mind of a black scientific racist and understand why blacks would help a movement that appears to be contrary to their community's and their own self-interest. George Schuyler says that a woman is nothing but "a child factory, as a cow is a milk factory and a hen an egg factory." He also states that there are "certain ingredients" that are necessary to produce a healthy child and that if these are missing then the "child will usually be an inferior product."[55] Human beings are nothing but products! It is unbelievable the callous disregard these people have for human life. W. E. B. Du Bois wanted blacks to "learn that among human races and groups, as among vegetables, quality and not mere quantity counts."[56] Elmer A. Carter was worried that the wrong blacks are having too many children, "Therein lies the danger, for Negroes who by virtue of their education and capacity are best able to rear children shrink from that responsibility and the Negro who, in addition to the handicaps of race and color, is shackled by mental and social incompetence serenely goes on his way bringing into the world children."[57] Du Bois also shared the sentiment the wrong kind of blacks were having children, "the mass of ignorant Negroes still breed carelessly and disastrously, so that the increase

---

[55] George S. Schulyer, "Quantity or Quality," *Birth Control Review* (June 1936): 165–66.

[56] Du Bois, "Black Folk and Birth Control," 166–67.

[57] Elmer A. Carter, "Eugenics for the Negro," *Birth Control Review* (June 1936): 169–70.

among Negroes, even more than among whites, is from that part of the population least intelligent and fit."[58] What you have read is how the black elites, who ally themselves with white eugenicist organizations, truly think of the black masses.

They also paint an extremely grim and pessimistic picture of life that doesn't seem to fit the reality. Only seventy years ago blacks lived as slaves; in 1932 they lived as freemen and were on the verge on gaining more of their constitutional rights. I think most people would see this as a hopeful situation. Of course, Du Bois and his friends are not concerned with painting an accurate picture of life or providing blacks with encouragement and hope. Their goal is to convince the blacks that are "shackled by mental and social incompetence," so it is better not to have any children. Schuyler seems to think that only morticians and prison wardens benefit from more black children, because that is where they are bound to end up. He wonders, "Why should the Negroes . . . continue to enrich the morticians and choke the jails with unwanted children?"[59] He

---

[58] Du Bois, "Black Folk and Birth Control," 166–67.
[59] Schulyer, "Quantity or Quality," 165–66.

also implores women to reject their innate maternal instincts and not have children, because "every child takes a great deal of vitality from even those mothers who are in the best of health"[60]

Planned Parenthood needed more front men than just black scholars, so they created the National Negro Advisory Council of the BCFA as a way to gain more influence in the black community. Sanger, using her charm, was able to convince many of the most prominent blacks of the day to join the council. The council received funding from Clarence Gamble, of the Proctor and Gamble family, and from the wife of advertising magnate Albert D. Lasker. Here is a partial list of some of the people who agreed to serve on the council:[61]

- Claude A. Barnett, Associated Negro Press

- Mary MacLeod Bethune, president, National Council of Negro Women, and special adviser to President Roosevelt

- Eugene K. Jones, executive secretary, National Urban League

---

[60] Ibid.
[61] Robert G. Marshall, *Blessed are the Barren: The Social Policy of Planned Parenthood* Ignatius Press, 1991, 19.

- L. Hollings Wood, president, National Urban League

- Frederick D. Patterson, president, Tuskegee Institute

- Charles D. Herbert, president, Morehouse College

- Rev. Adam Clayton Powell, U.S. congressman.

The council provided more "black cover" for eugenics. Some members may have joined the council because they considered it an honor to be invited to join a group of such prominent people. But, don't be mistaken, not all members were dupes joining the council to just rub elbows with the rich and famous. The words of board member Dr. Dorothy B. Ferebee, president of the nation's largest black sorority, show that she knew full well the intended goal of birth control and the benefit of having fellow blacks serve as the face of the eugenics movement. She stated that one of their "most difficult obstacles" was the belief that birth control was "motivated by a clever bit of machination to persuade them to commit race suicide."[62] She believed the best way to calm peoples' fears was to "utilize Negro

---

[62] Ibid.

professionals," because they "would not be suspected of the intent to eliminate the race."[63]

Planned Parenthood did not limit its propaganda effort to scholarly journals and America's black elites. It also sought to change the attitudes of the masses by spreading its propaganda in the mainstream media. In mainstream media outlets, fearmongering was one of Planned Parenthood's preferred methods. The organization would send press releases to black newspapers to print. On March 29, 1947, the *Pittsburgh Courier*, one of the nation's leading black newspapers, printed a Planned Parenthood press release as if it was an article written by a *Courier* journalist. The article ominously asked the reader, "Did you know that Negro mothers die at twice the rate of white mothers? Did you know that Negro babies die one and half times faster than white babies? Did you know that before their first birthday some 22,000 Negro babies are dead?" The article then boldly declares in all capitals that, "PPFA HAS THE ANSWERS." PPFA stands for the Planned

---

[63] Ibid., 20.

Parenthood Federation of America. A local Pittsburgh priest with a black congregation read this article and sent a fiery letter to the editor wondering, "Why the colored press should advocate a practice that will decimate the colored race is beyond me."[64] The priest asked the obvious question: If it is true that black babies die at twice the rate of white babies, then shouldn't efforts be made to improve the conditions for black people instead of trying to decrease the amount of black babies born. Of course Planned Parenthood isn't interesting improving the conditions of blacks. Its only interest is in the total decimation of the black population.

In addition to placing propaganda in the mainstream media, Planned Parenthood believed, the best approach was to reach blacks through the churches by hiring "'colored ministers, preferably with social service backgrounds, and with engaging personalities' to travel the South and propagandize for birth control."[65] "The most successful educational approach to the Negro is through a religious appeal," Sanger wrote, because,

[64] Rev. Francis Donland, Letter. *Pittsburgh Courier*, 19 April 1947.
[65] Gordon, *Woman's Body, Woman's Right,* 332.

"We do not want word to go out that we want to exterminate the Negro population and the minister is the man who can straighten out that idea if it ever occurs to any of their rebellious members."[66]

Sanger worked tirelessly trying to receive endorsements and support from black leaders. She wrote everyone in *Colored Who's Who* and called on as many prominent blacks as humanly possible. The way she convinced skeptical Reverend J. T. Braun, editor in chief of the National Baptist Convention's Sunday School Publishing Board in Nashville, Tennessee, is illustrative of her methods. Braun expressed his wariness of birth control to Sanger. "The very idea of such a thing [birth control] has always held the greatest hatred and contempt in my mind. . . . I am hesitant to give my full endorsement of this idea, until you send me, perhaps, some more convincing literature on the subject."[67] Sanger sent him pamphlets that were praised by another black minister and convinced him that her

[66] Ibid., 332–33

[67] Tanya L. Green, *"The Negro Project: Margaret Sanger's Eugenic Plan for Black Americans,"* http://www.citizenreviewonline.org/special_issues/population/the_negro_pro ject.htm, 10 May 2001.

interest in birth control was only out of concern for black people's health, particularly infant mortality. In this manner she was able to convince Braun that she had nothing but noble intentions. Braun must have thought why would so many other blacks support her if she did not have good intentions? He must have thought she is such nice lady; most whites want nothing to do with blacks. Braun eventually capitulated and reversed his previously anti-birth control opinion and allowed his church to be used for birth control propaganda sessions.[68]

In addition to getting ministers to act as front men, Planned Parenthood hired black doctors to provide birth control services. The doctors would only be allowed to use Planned Parenthood's funds for birth control, never for any other health-related matters. Gamble made it clear that he did not care at all about the well-being of blacks when he informed the public health director of South Carolina that Planned Parenthood's money should be used for birth control and not be "diluted with a lot of general health work."[69]

---

[68] Ibid.
[69] Gordon, *Woman's Body, Woman's Right*, 333.

Blacks would appear to be in charge, but it was merely an illusion. Dr Lydia DeVilbiss pulled funding from an all-black birth control clinic in Miami because they were not following her directives as much as she would have liked. In a letter she wondered whether, "southern darkies can ever be entrusted with such a clinic. Our experience causes to doubt their ability to work except under white supervision."[70] Overall, Planned Parenthood had success in their doctor outreach program. It was reported that in Nashville, Tennessee, 80 percent of "low intelligence" blacks would use birth control after receiving instructions.[71]

George Grant, Planned Parenthood researcher and historian, explains their tactics this way:

> The entire operation then was a ruse—a manipulative attempt to get Blacks to cooperate in their own elimination.

---

[70] Ibid. 330.
[71] George Grant, *Grand Illusions: The Legacy of Planned Parenthood* Highland Books, 1998 19.

The program's genocidal intentions were carefully camouflaged beneath several layers of condescending social service rhetoric and organizational expertise. Like the citizens of Hamelin, lured into captivity by the sweet serenades of the Pied Piper[72]

It may seem counterintuitive to hire the most conservative and educated members of the community to lead blacks on the path to self-destruction, but by befriending the leadership of the black community, they squashed any effective opposition to their plans of genocide. Most blacks expect racists to wear white hoods and to show open hostility towards blacks. These racists do exist, but the more insidious racists are the ones wearing three-piece suits with gentlemanly manners and charm. They operate like a con artist that builds a rapport to gain the trust and confidence of his victims only to betray that trust, but unlike a con artist, it is not your money they are after, it is your life.

---

[72] Ibid., 41.

Chapter 5: Promoting Birth Control

So far I have described Planned Parenthood's propaganda efforts with, primarily, the elites of black America. These social engineering efforts are necessary because they lay the groundwork for Planned Parenthood's ultimate objective, the elimination of the black race. Its attack plan can be thought of as a two-pronged pincer attack. One pincer attacks from above and is aimed at the elites. The goal is to convince elites that Planned Parenthood and eugenics are not their enemies but their friends. The eugenicists know that the most effective resistance comes from the elites of society, and this is why the elites must be neutralized. The rich and the educated have the knowledge and resources to launch an effective counterattack. For example, look at the American Revolution. Our Founding Fathers were not poor and uneducated; they were the richest, most educated, and most prominent members of society. They had the money to print revolutionary pamphlets and the education to write effective tracts against the king and they were men of prominence, so when they spoke out against King George, people listened. The words of a doctor or a successful businessman carry more weight with the general public than the same words spoken by a simple laborer. By co-opting the black elites, Planned Parenthood was nullifying any true resistance.

The second arm of Planned Parenthood's attack was attacks from below. Here is where Planned Parenthood does the dirty work of exterminating the black race. Some of the tactics in this attack plan are birth control, sterilizations, and abortions.

Most of Planned Parenthood's activist works goes undocumented and unreported by the mainstream media. It often targets poor neighborhoods where the people don't have the means, the time, or the ability to mount a resistance. Usually, the only educated people in poor neighborhoods are ministers. If resistance to Planned Parenthood were to take place, it would most likely come from the ministers. Ministers have the education, leadership, and communication skills to organize the community, write letters to the editor, and possibly find a sympathetic journalist to report on Planned Parenthood's activities. This is why Margaret Sanger's following comment is so salient: "The most successful educational approach to the Negro is through a religious appeal. We do not want word to go out that we want to exterminate the Negro population and the minister is the man who can straighten out that idea if it ever occurs to any of their rebellious members."[73]

In Pittsburgh, Planned Parenthood faced rare resistance from the local community. A big part of the reason it faced resistance is because Pittsburgh has a large black Catholic population. It is harder for Planned Parenthood to buy a Catholic priest then it is to buy a Protestant minister because of the Catholic Church's hierarchal structure. Every priest must answer to his bishop, so Planned Parenthood would have to buy the Bishop. Most protestant denominations don't have a rigid hierarchal structure like the Catholic Church. . The downside of having a hierarchal structure is that if you can control the Bishop, you control all the priests under him. In Pittsburgh,

---

[73] Gordon, *Woman's Body, Woman's Right*, 332–33

there was a white Catholic priest of a local congregation in a black Pittsburgh neighborhood, Father Charles Owen Rice, that they did not control and, more importantly, they also did not control his Bishop. When Father Rice learned of Planned Parenthood's activities, he decided to fight and expose them. Luckily, Father Rice had allies. Not only did he have the support of his Bishop but he had the support Dr. Charles Greenlee, a black doctor and chair of the medical committee of the Pittsburgh branch of the NAACP chapter, and William "Bouie" Haden, a Black Nationalist and local community leader. These three men formed an unlikely alliance to try to prevent and expose birth control programs they felt were a plot to decimate the black poor.

Because Planned Parenthood faced resistance in Pittsburgh, many of its activities there were unusually well documented, which provides a valuable insight into Planned Parenthood's tactics and methods. During the John F. Kennedy administration, Planned Parenthood received an infusion of new federal funding that allowed it to greatly increase its reach into

America's black communities. In Pittsburgh, it began opening birth control clinics in Pittsburgh's black neighborhoods but not in its white neighborhoods. Planned Parenthood not only opened new birth control clinics, but it also established a home visitor program. The program sent workers to educate women, including single women, on the benefits of birth control. The workers showed the women pro-birth control propaganda films and offered the women free contraceptives. They even paid for babysitters so young mothers could go to the clinic to get their birth control devices, and if they couldn't leave the house, someone would be sent to their house to give them their pills.[74]

Planned Parenthood claimed that it was only concerned about the health of poor black women. Dr. Greenlee, Bouie Haden, and Fr. Rice did not believe that Planned Parenthood had benign motivations behind its actions. They felt the true nefarious goal of these programs was to commit genocide by reducing the black birthrate. And they were right according to the United Nations Convention of Genocide in 1948 that stated

---

74 John Woodford, "Birth Control: White Man's Heaven?" *Muhamad Speaks* (24 January 1969): 7–8.

"imposing measures intended to prevent births within the group" is one way of committing genocide. They decided to warn people and tried to publicize Planned Parenthood's operations through the media. "Planned Parenthood & the OEO (Office of Economic Opportunity) have a humming pill mill in Negro poverty areas. They send lay people around with all manner of contraceptives from door to door to Negroes," is how Fr. Rice described the program.[75] Dr. Greenlee felt the films shown to the women were designed to convince them to stop having babies, and he called the home visitor program nothing more than a "session of brain-washing."[76]

It seemed strange to many that the same government spending millions of dollars for free contraceptives and birth control propaganda does not pay for a man's hospital bills if he breaks a leg, does not pay for medication if a person gets sick, and does not pay for a babysitter when a young mother needs one to get to school or work. As Dr. Charles Greenlee put it, the

---

75 Simone M. Caron, "Birth Control and the Black Community in The 1960s: Genocide Or Power Politics?" *Journal of Social History* (Spring 1998): 556.
76 Ibid.

"power structure won't spend a dime to kill the rats that eat up your babies, but they'll spend thousands to make sure you can't have any babies."[77] To Greenlee, Haden, and Rice the evidence was obvious that the government and Planned Parenthood were launching a systematic plan to lower the black birthrate that amounted to genocide.

Planned Parenthood reacted the way it usually does when confronted about its activities. It will deny all charges and claim that it is acting out of concern for the poor. In Pittsburgh Planned Parenthood expressed disbelief that anyone could even accuse it of something so awful, saying that it was "'shocked' because the accusations 'were so completely remote from our philosophy' that they believed that 'somewhere along the line, a deep misunderstanding of our program and services had crept in.'"[78] Planned Parenthood claimed that its only motivation was to educate the poor on the benefits of birth control and to provide birth control to those who wanted it. Although the observations made by Father Rice and others may appear

---

77 Ibid., 555.
78 Ibid, 557.

sinister, they all had a simple explanation. The home visitor program's only purpose was to educate women on the benefits of child spacing. Planned Parenthood launched its own publicity campaign to convince the public that goals were nothing but benign and that allegations of genocide were only the ravings of paranoid conspiracy theorists.

Planned Parenthood public relations campaign did not convince the Catholic Bishops of Pennsylvania, and on June 20, 1966, they placed a full-page ad in sixty Pennsylvanian newspapers accusing Planned Parenthood and the federal government of trying to reduce the black population with taxpayer-funded birth control programs. Below is a passage from the advertisement:

> While no word appears in the proposal to indicate that this augmented birth prevention policy is aimed at Negro citizens in Pennsylvania, it is widely, though covertly, stated by birth prevention proponents both in and out of government that a significant "benefit" of

these programs would be their supposedly resulting check upon the expanding Negro populations in our major cities. Discussion of such benefits is not infrequently accompanied with such racist phrases as "limiting the number of undesirables" and with defamatory innuendo concerning alleged Negro "traits" and the dangers of Negro "proliferation."[79]

Dr. Greenlee was able to convince the Pittsburgh branch of the NAACP to issue a statement that Planned Parenthood's clinics were behaving "without moral responsibility to the black race and become an instrument of genocide for the Negro people."[80] The Pittsburgh branch, not surprisingly, received no support from the national offices of the NAACP, which was and still is securely in Planned Parenthood's pocket. It is not surprising that Dr. Greenlee found and noted that, "I've talked

---

[79] "Statement of the Catholic Bishops of Pennsylvania on State Sponsored Birth Control Programs," *Philadelphia Inquirer*, June 20, 1966.
[80] "Negroes Criticize Family Planners," *New York Times*, December 17, 1967.

to some Black men who support the extermination of poor—

that is most—Black people too."[81]

Many of the blacks who work for Planned Parenthood
are well-intentioned people who are under the illusion that they
are actually helping people. They are just useful idiots. Mrs.
Ruby Wyatt Evans learned the hard way that Planned
Parenthood only needs blacks for cover. She learned that
Planned Parenthood's black employees are expendable once
they are no longer useful in helping Planned Parenthood achieve
their genocidal objectives. She was suspended from Planned
Parenthood when she told women that they "didn't have to take
the pills if they did not desire."[82]

In Cook County, Illinois, Planned Parenthood's efforts
were very successful in lowering the black birthrate. Hospitals
in the county began to show new mothers pro-birth control
propaganda films. These films were shown to the mothers right
after they had given birth and before the mothers had a chance

---

[81] Woodford, "Birth Control: White Man's Heaven?" *Muhamad Speaks* 24
Jan. 1969: 37.
[82] "Dispute on 'Pill,' Race Hits U.S.," *Pittsburgh Courier* December 30,
1967.

to see their new baby. The movies would "tell the mother that life would be better for her and her family if she would enter the birth control program. They try to make her sorry she even had the little baby which has just arrived."[83] This program reduced births in the county by 10 percent from 1968 to 1969, but hospitals in predominately white neighborhoods in the county only saw a 1.8 percent decline in births.[84] Dr. Robert Freeark, medical chief of the Cook County Hospital, said that the decline in births was "almost entirely" a result of Planned Parenthood efforts and family planning clinics.[85]

A black official with the Office of Economic Opportunity (OEO) told *Muhammad Speaks* that the government, in conjunction with Planned Parenthood, had, using the theory of cognitive dissonance, developed brainwashing techniques to convince blacks to use birth control. The centerpiece of their strategy was to always use female black birth control field workers to invite other young women to their

---

[83] Ogun Kakanfo, "What Happens When Birth Control Succeeds? Part 2," *Muhammad Speaks* (11 July 1969): 15.
[84] Ibid.
[85] Ibid.

house for coffee. The field worker would explain the benefits of birth control. Pro-birth control films would be shown and young women who are already on birth control would be invited to speak about how much better the pill has made their life. [86]

Planned Parenthood still uses clever marketing, or if you prefer, brainwashing methods, to get blacks to have fewer children. It now gives away coupons and pop records and sponsors dances to get women in their clinics.[87] In Akron, Ohio, Planned Parenthood put bags containing a coupon for a $5 McDonalds' gift certificate and twelve free condoms redeemable at one of three Planned Parenthood clinics on the doorknobs in poor black neighborhoods. Among the items found in the bag were a condom key chain, literature on contraception, pen, mirror, and notepad. All items had Planned Parenthood's number imprinted on them. Planned Parenthood admits that only certain neighborhoods were targeted with the promotional campaign, and of course it claims it is a mere

---

[86] Ogun Kakanfo, "How to Brainwash Women into Swallowing the Pill," *Muhammad Speaks* (8 August 1969): 7, 16, 37.
[87] Grant, *Grand Illusions*, 112.

coincidence that those neighborhoods happened to be black. Fr. Richard Welch of Human Life International commented, "Having sprung from the racist dreams of a woman determined to apply abortion and contraception to eugenics and ethnic cleansing, Planned Parenthood remains true to the strategy today"[88]

Planned Parenthood not only has neighborhood-based clinics but it also now puts clinics right inside public schools in an attempt to reach people when they are most impressionable. These clinics distribute free contraception devices and provide information on abortion. Of the first 100 of these school-based clinics that were opened, none were put in all-white schools. All were in schools with a Hispanic or black population.[89] Louisiana state representative Sharon Weston Broome learned firsthand about the true motivations of those who wanted to place birth control clinics in her district's black schools. In the late 1990s, Baton Rouge officials were debating a proposal to

---

[88] Lisa Ing, "Condom Giveaway Based on Profiling, Pro-Lifers Contend," *Washington Times* 31 July 2000.
[89] Grant, *Grand Illusions*, 109.

put birth control clinics in the area's black schools. When Representative Sharon Weston Broome urged that the clinics be put in white schools as well, the proposal was "dropped immediately."[90] In 1986 a group of thirteen black clergy men sued the city of Chicago to stop the distribution of free condoms at DuSable High School. Rev. Hiram Crawford asked, "If these clinics are so good for black kids, why don't they put them in white areas? It's a form of genocide"[91]

Planned Parenthood's own internal statistics prove that it is targeting young blacks. In 1980 black teenagers represented 44 percent of all teenage visits to Planned Parenthood clinics. [92] This is an extremely disproportionate representation considering blacks were only about 12 percent of the population. A 1976 study published by the Alan Guttamacher Institute, the research area of Planned Parenthood, bragged on how successful family

---

[90] Tanya L. Green, "The Negro Project: Margaret Sanger's Eugenic Plan for Black Americans,"
http://www.citizenreviewonline.org/special_issues/population/the_negro_pro ject.htm, 10 May 2001.
[91] John Leo, "Sex and Schools Aids and the Surgeon General Add a New Urgency to an Old Debate," *Time Magazine*, 24 November 1986.
[92] Laurie Schwab Zabin and Samuel D. Clark, "Why the Delay: A Study of Teenage Family Planning Clinic Patients," *Family Planning Perspectives* (September–October 1981).

planning was at reducing the fertility of poor women. The study was especially pleased that family planning was projected to reduce the fertility of black woman at a greater rate than white women. The study predicted that if all poor white women were enrolled in family planning, fertility would be reduced by 54 births per 1,000, but "among black wives 20–29, the program effects were even more striking—a projected reduction of 97 per 1,000 . . . might be expected."[93]

Birth control by using contraceptives is a slow method of committing genocide. One of the problems with birth control is that it is not permanent. A woman could practice birth control for a number of years and then get married and have twelve children. It is for this reason that the eugenicists also use more permanent methods like sterilization. Sterilizations were not as popular with the American public as birth control, so the eugenicists' sterilization efforts have always been more hidden. Eugenicists began lobbying state legislatures for bills requiring

---

[93] "Subsidized Family planning Program Has Helped U.S. Low-Income Women to Reduce Their Fertility," *International Family planning Digest* (June 1976): 7–8.

the forced sterilization of prisoners, the mentally impaired, and the poor. Early attempts to pass sterilization laws in Michigan and Pennsylvania failed, but eventually, by 1914 some sort of forced sterilization laws were passed in twelve states.[94] There was no public support for these laws, and even the Eugenics Section of the American Breeders Association admitted that a "very small energetic group of enthusiasts" were responsible for the legislation and that "public sentiment demanding action was absent."[95] The sterilization movement, by the eugenicists' own admission, was not a grassroots movement but a movement of small cabal of elites.

They did face resistance, and Virginia's law was challenged in the courts. In 1927, in the *Buck vs. Bell* case, the Supreme Court upheld Virginia's forced sterilization law in an 8 to 1 decision. Chief Justice Oliver Wendell Holmes wrote the majority opinion for the court. He wrote, "It is better for all the world, if instead of waiting to execute degenerate offspring for

---

[94] Paul Lombardo, "Eugenic Sterilization Laws," http://www.eugenicsarchive.org/html/eugenics/essay8text.html.
[95] Black, *War against the Weak*, 69.

crime, or to let them starve for their imbecility, society can prevent those who are manifestly unfit from continuing their kind."

He finished his opinion ruling that Carrie Buck, a young white woman who did not want to be sterilized, must be forced to have the operation with the frank statement, "Three generations of imbeciles are enough." This decision launched a surge in sterilizations, because doctors and bureaucrats had been hesitant before to perform and allow sterilizations because the constitutionality of the laws was always suspect. States now emboldened with the stamp of approval from the Supreme Court began to liberally sterilize people. A total of 35,878 people were sterilized from 1907 to 1940, and 30,000 came after the Buck decision[96]. North Carolina established a eugenics board to recommend people for sterilization. From 1929 to 1974 at least 7,600 people were sterilized and 60 percent of them were black.[97] St. Agnes, a historic black hospital, played an

---

[96] Ibid., 123.
[97] Janell Ross, "Eugenics Bill Is Back on the Table; Womble Pushes for Victim Stipend," *The News and Observer*, June 10, 2006.

active role in the sterilizations, and black doctors also recommended other blacks to undergo forced sterilizations.[98]

When the authorities were unable to force involuntary sterilizations, other coercive methods were used. In New Bern, North Carolina, in 1965 an eighteen-year-old unwed mother, Nial Ruth Cox, was told that she must undergo a permanent sterilization procedure or else her family would lose their welfare benefits. She was also lied to and told the procedure would only be temporary.[99] Miss Cox was not the only case of young woman agreeing to be sterilized because of threats and trickery. Dorothy Waters was told by her doctor that he would not deliver her baby unless she agreed to undergo sterilization. Dr. Clovis Pierce of the Aiken County Hospital in South Carolina told her, "Listen here, young lady, this is my tax money paying for this baby and I'm tired of paying for illegitimate children."[100] Many other women in Aiken County

---

[98] Janell Ross, "Historic Black Hospital Tied to Sterilization Program," *The News and Observer*, May 14, 2006.
[99] Jack Slater "Sterilization: Newest Threat to the Poor," *Ebony* (October 1973): 150–56.
[100] Robert G. Weisbord, *Genocide?: Birth Control and the Black American* Greenwood Press, 1975, 162.

reported similar experiences. A $1.5 million lawsuit was filed by two women against the county alleging that Dr. Pierce threatened to terminate their welfare benefits and not attend to the woman during and after labor.[101]

Dr. Pierce sterilized eighteen women, seventeen of them black, before his actions became public. The South Carolina establishment came to Dr. Pierce's aid. The Aiken County Medical Society refused any sanctions on the doctor and praised him for his "professional integrity and competence."[102] The South Carolina State Legislature passed a special motion in December of 1973, just for Dr. Pierce, reasserting that doctors were presumed innocent. One state legislator, Cecil Collins, expressed his support for Dr. Pierce by saying that welfare mothers should be sterilized the first time they have an out-of-wedlock child.[103] This was not the only place women were pressured in to being sterilized. Dr. Bernard Rosenfeld claimed to have firsthand knowledge of a dozen cases were women were

---

[101] Ibid., 163.
[102] Ibid., 165.
[103] Ibid.

asked to consent to sterilization minutes before undergoing a Caesarian.[104] There are reports of similar incidents in the Boston City Hospital and the Los Angeles County Hospital.[105]

In Alabama the authorities didn't wait for a young woman to become pregnant before trying to sterilize her. Two sisters in Montgomery, Minnie Relf, age fourteen, and Mary Alice, age twelve, were tricked into being sterilized. Representatives from the federally financed Montgomery Community Action Agency (MCAC) contacted their mother and told her that her daughters needed some shots. The mother, who was unable to read or write, put her X on consent form, thinking that authorities were only looking after her interests. The shots turned out to Depo Provera a drug that temporarily prevents pregnancy. Representatives from Planned Parenthood and MCAC came by a second time and told the mother that she should sign another form to continue the shots. The form was not for a continuation of the shots but a sterilization authorization form. Mrs. Relf put an X on the form and her two

---

[104] Ibid., 153.
[105] Ibid., 153–54.

daughters were sterilized. While the two sisters were in the hospital, Planned Parenthood workers came to the house and tried to convince their older sister, Katie, age sixteen, to receive the same shots. When Katie told the workers she wanted to have children in the future, they told her, "I don't think you need any." Katie locked herself in her room until the workers left. The father, Lonnie Relf, found out about the sterilizations when a social worker investigated and told him what happened to his daughters. He filed a $1 million lawsuit. Crelia Dixon of Planned Parenthood responded to the lawsuit by stating, "We talked to them (speaking about the young girls) about other possible alternatives that they could possibly use," and they agreed for the sterilization operation.[106] At least eighty young girls were sterilized in this manner between 1972 and 1973.[107] These are not isolated incidents, even Naomi T. Gray, a onetime vice president of Planned Parenthood, stated she personally knew of a "substantial" number of black women who had been

---

[106] "Black Girls Tricked into Sterilization," *The Black Panther* (7 July 1973): 5.
[107] Slater, 150–56, and Drummond B. Ayres, "Sterilizing the Poor— Exploring Motives and Methods," *New York Times*, 8 July 1973.

tricked into have sterilization operations.[108] Because of these and other efforts, the sterilization rate among blacks is 45 percent higher than it is among whites.[109]

Planned Parenthood would like to have the practice of forced sterilizations widely accepted and commonplace. A March 11, 1969, memorandum written by Frederick S. Jaffe of Planned Parenthood entitled "Activities Relevant to the Study of Population Policy" called for "compulsory sterilization for those who have already had two children."[110]

Planned Parenthood is known as a "liberal" organization, so they are not as open and vocal in advocating forced sterilization as conservatives. Conservatives can be more outspoken about their belief in sterilization, and during the 1960s and 1970s, conservative leaders were upfront in their advocacy of sterilizing welfare mothers. A law that passed the Mississippi house in 1964 made it a felony, punishable by 1 to 3 years in prison, to have a second out-of-wedlock child. The

---

[108] Weisbord, *Genocide?*, 152.
[109] Grant, *Grand Illusions*, 111.
[110] Ibid., 55.

person could get out of doing time if they agreed to be sterilized.[111] Similar measures were proposed in Tennessee, South Carolina, Illinois, and Ohio legislatures.[112] In January of 1971, Vice President Spiro Agnew asked who was going to tell the welfare mother, "We're very sorry but we will not be able to allow you to have more children."[113] Nobel Peace Prize winner William Shockley proposed a sterilization bonus plan of paying people a $1,000 to be sterilized for every I.Q. point below 100. So a person with a 70 I.Q. would receive $30,000 to be sterilized.[114] Recently an Ohio elected official, the Geauga County commissioner, has called for sterilizing all welfare parents.[115]

Chapter 6: Promoting Abortions

[111] Weisbord, *Genocide?*, 141–42.
[112] Ibid., 144–47.
[113] Ibid., 48.
[114] Stefan Kühl, *The Nazi Connection: Eugenics, American Racism, and German National Socialism* Oxford University Press, 1994 7.
[115] Michael O'Malley, "The Longest Shot for Governor, Geauga County Commissioner Advocates for Sterilization," *Plain Dealer*, 27 April 2006.

Although birth control and sterilizations are ugly methods of committing genocide, their most deadly method is abortion. Until the cultural revolution of the 1960s, the overwhelming majority of Americans viewed abortion as an anathema. Margaret Sanger was advised by Havelock Ellis not to advocate abortion because it was too controversial, but instead to state that birth control was a means of eliminating abortion. Margaret Sanger followed his advice and no longer fought for, in her words a woman's "right to destroy" but instead for a woman's "right to create or not create a new life."[116] Ellis knew if Planned Parenthood were publicly in favor of abortion it would destroy their credibility and effectiveness. Even as late as 1963 Planned Parenthood was publicly against abortion and put out a pamphlet that described the differences between abortion and birth control in this way: "Is birth control an abortion? Definitely not. An abortion kills the life of a baby after it has begun. It is dangerous to your life and health. It may

---

[116] Drogin, *Margaret Sanger*, 87.

make you sterile so that when you want a child you cannot have it. Birth control merely post-pones the beginning of life."[117]

It is interesting to note that now pro-abortion advocates claim that a fetus is not a human life; so therefore, it is perfectly OK to kill it. The early eugenicists were not at all confused on whether or not a fetus is a human life. They understood a fetus is a human life, and if it was a genetically inferior human, they wanted to kill it.

On January 22, 1973, the Supreme Court in the landmark *Roe v. Wade* decision accomplished what could never have been accomplished through the democratic process; it legalized abortion. By this time Planned Parenthood was the most vocal and well-funded supporter of abortion. Planned Parenthood began to open abortion clinics and now is the nation's leading abortion provider.[118] Since this decision, more than twelve million black babies have been aborted, many times

---

[117] Dr. and Mrs. J. C. Willke, "Why Can't We Love them Both?" http://www.abortionfacts.com/online_books/love_them_both/why_cant_we_love_them_both_42.asp.
[118] Planned Parenthood Press Release, "Clinics Stay Open," http://www.plannedparenthood.org/news-articles-press/politics-policy-issues/clinics-5789.htm, 8 March 2006.

more than the 3,445 blacks estimated to have been lynched between 1882 and the 1960s.[119]

Not only have an incredible number of black babies been aborted, but black babies also are more likely to be aborted than whites. According to Planned Parenthood's research arm, the Alan Guttmacher Institute, in 2002 43 percent of black pregnancies ended in abortion compared to only 18 percent of white pregnancies.[120] Blacks make up only 12 percent of the population yet account for 35 percent of all abortions.[121] In some states the disparity is even starker. In Mississippi blacks account for 37 percent of the population but for 73 percent of the abortions[122], and in Pennsylvania blacks account for 10 percent of the population but for 45 percent of abortions.[123] The federal government's Center for Disease Control and Prevention

---

[119] Anthony Bradley, "Abortion by Race," *World Magazine* (19 February 2005)

[120] Catherine Tsai, "Beauprez Apologizes for Wrong Abortion Statistic," *The Associated Press State & Local Wire*, 31 August 2006.

[121] Bradley, Abortion by Race,"

[122] Ibid.

[123] Steven Ertelt, "Crisis Pregnancy Centers Eye Inner Cities to Help Black Women Avoid Abortion," http://www.lifenews.com/nat2518.html, 21 Aug 2006.

data shows that the abortion rate among blacks is three times higher than the abortion rate among whites.[124]

It is not surprising that blacks are aborting their babies at a much greater rate than whites considering that Planned Parenthood and other abortion providers target blacks and others living in poor urban communities. Ninety-four percent of abortion mills are located in urban areas[125] and 90 percent of women who obtain abortions live in urban areas.[126] A study by the American Life League found that the higher the percentage of minorities in a city the greater the number of abortion clinics. They looked at fifteen cities with a minority population greater than 25 percent and fifteen cities with a minority population less than 25 percent. In the cities with a higher concentration of minorities there were five abortion clinics per million people but only three clinics per million people in the cities with a small minority population.[127]

---

[124] Tammie Smith, "Few Black Voices Heard on Abortion," *Richmond Times Dispatch*, 3 March 2005.
[125] Steve Jordahl, "Pregnancy Centers Go Downtown," http://www.family.org/cforum/fnif/news/a0041720.cfm, 22 August 2006.
[126] David Crary, "Pro-life on Murder Row," *Washington Times* 22 Aug 2006.
[127] American Life League, *Pro-Life Activist's Encyclopedia* http://www.ewtn.com/library/PROLENC/ENCYC078.HTM, CHAPTER

Just placing abortion clinics in black neighborhoods is not enough. Planned Parenthood needed a plan to get blacks to go in to those clinics and abort their babies. Planned Parenthood has essentially used the tactics and strategies laid out in Margaret Sanger's Negro Project. As Sanger noted in the Negro Project, "The most successful educational approach to the Negro is through a religious appeal. We do not want word to go out that we want to exterminate the Negro population and the minister is the man who can straighten out that if it ever occurs to any of their more rebellious members"[128]

Planned Parenthood has black ministers act as front men and Judas goats to persuade people to have abortions. It is not difficult to figure out who those black front men today are. The most visible are Rev. Jesse Jackson and Rev. Al Sharpton. Both men have been appointed as the leaders and spokesmen for black America by the media. Why would the media appoint these two men? It is not because they have large and vibrant congregations. Even though both men claim to be ministers,

78—ABORTION: THE RACIST'S MOST DEVASTATING WEAPON.
[128] Gordon, *Woman's Body, Woman's Right*, 332–33.

neither one has a church. Now if you or I went around calling ourselves ministers, but didn't preside over a church, we would get strange looks. But not Al and Jesse; they are media darlings, and they hobnob with the liberal establishment. It is clear that these men are not where they are because of grassroots support from below but because they were selected from above by the elites. Not only do they not have a church but they also have little popular support in the black community. Polls show only 15 percent of blacks consider Jesse Jackson the "most important black leader" and 2 percent picked Al Sharpton.[129] Their power and support comes from the establishment, not the common man.

Al Sharpton has a completely irrational position on abortion. In his book *Al on America*, he states that, "Life begins when a sperm meets the egg, and that only God should decide whether to take a life." But in the same book he contradicts himself and declares that if he were president, he would only

---

[129] Sean Alfano, "Poll: Jesse Jackson, Rice Top Blacks," http://www.cbsnews.com/stories/2006/02/15/national/main1321719.shtml, 2 February 2006.

appoint Supreme Court justices who are for giving "women the right to choose whether or not they will have an abortion."[130] How can one believe that life begins at conception but also believe that life deserves no protection and can be lawfully killed? No matter how irrational his position, Al Sharpton is always ready to provide "black cover" for the establishment whenever they are criticized on abortion. He is handsomely rewarded for being a Judas goat. He gets invited to upscale Planned Parenthood-sponsored dinners with the liberal elite and lists among his generous financial backers left-wing celebrities like Barbara Streisand.[131] Al Sharpton knows the minute he advocates a pro-life position is the minute his donations from the liberal elite stop and his name will no longer appear in papers.

Jesse Jackson's pro-abortion position is even more perplexing than Sharpton's. Jesse Jackson was born out of wedlock. According to Jackson his mother choose not to follow

---

[130] Paul Nowak, "Al Sharpton's Actions Wouldn't Match Words on Abortion," http://www.catholicexchange.com/vm/PFarticle.asp?vm_id=31&art_id=21474&sec_id=40902, 3 December 2003.
[131] Ibid.

the advice of her doctor, who told her to have an abortion. Because he was almost aborted, he had, like most ministers, a stridently anti-abortion position.[132] In a 1977 letter Jackson expresses his strong pro-life position: "Human beings cannot give or create life by themselves, it is really a gift from God. Therefore, one does not have the right to take away (through abortion) that which he does not have the ability to give." [133] And, "Those advocates of taking life prior to birth do not call it killing or murder, they call it abortion. They further never talk about aborting a baby because that would imply something human. Rather, they talk about aborting the fetus. Fetus sounds less than human and therefore can be justified."[134]

God creates life and only God can take life. It seems simple, but I guess God no longer creates life because now Jesse Jackson is strongly pro-abortion. Why the flip-flop? Jackson has given no answer for his change in his positions. But

---

[132] Colman McCarthy, "Jackson's Reversal on Abortion," *Washington Post*, 21 May 1988.

[133] Ibid.

[134] Jesse Jackson, "How We Respect Life Is the Over-Riding Moral Issue," *Right to Life News*, http://swiss.csail.mit.edu/~rauch/nvp/consistent/jackson.html, 1977 January.

it is interesting to note that he changed his position right before his 1988 presidential campaign. It is well known that being pro-abortion is a necessity for any Democrat running for president. Pro-life Democratic representative Bart Stupak says his pro-life position has cost him financial support from the liberal elite.[135] If you are pro-life and a Democrat running for president, the Democratic establishment will actively oppose you and you will have no shot of winning the nomination. So Jesse was given a choice to follow conscience and principles or to satisfy his ambition. Jesse Jackson sold his soul and picked glory and power over principles. So the Jesse of 1977 said, "Some argue, suppose the woman does not want to have the baby. They say the very fact that she does not want the baby means that the psychological damage to the child is enough to abort the baby. I disagree. The solution to that problem is not to kill the innocent baby but to deal with her values and her attitude toward life— that which has allowed her not to want the baby." Now he says,

---

[135] Patricia Zapor, "Pro-life Democrats Describe Lonely Role, but See Improvements,"
http://www.catholicnews.com/data/stories/cns/0404122.htm, 28 July 2004.

"Women must have freedom of choice over what to do over their bodies."[136] Jesse used to say he thought, "If one accepts the position that life is private, and therefore you have the right to do with it as you please, one must also accept the conclusion of that logic. That was the premise of slavery. You could not protest the existence or treatment of slaves on the plantation because that was private and therefore outside your right to be concerned." Now he says, "it is not right to impose private, religious and moral positions on public policy."[137]

As more and more black people learn the true nature of the abortion movement, more blacks are adopting a pro-life position. According to a 2004 Zogby poll, 68 percent of blacks are now pro-life.[138] This makes abortion just one of many issues (illegal immigration, homosexual marriage, school choice, and prayer are others) that the black establishment is out of touch with majority of blacks. The establishment is definitely nervous that they are losing control over black people. Al Sharpton and

---

[136] McCarthy, "Jackson's Reversal On Abortion."
[137] Ibid.
[138] Steven Ertelt, "New Poll: Majority of Americans, Blacks, Students Pro-Life on Abortion," http://www.lifenews.com/nat474.html, 26 April 2004.

Jesse Jackson sponsored a conference to criticize black churches, calling them to stop focusing on moral issues like homosexual marriage and abortion and to concentrate on the Democratic agenda. Bishop Harry Jackson Jr., a democrat and a pastor of a church with more than three thousand parishioners, responded to Jackson and Sharpton's criticism by saying, "There is a new black church that Al and Jesse don't speak to, and they are threatened by the new black mega churches and their pastors; and they tend to talk about us as if we are just uppity Negroes, asking 'why can't they just fall in line?'"[139]

Jackson and Sharpton are not the only front men used to "straighten out" the more "rebellious members" who oppose the extermination of the black race. In 1996 the Religious Coalition for Reproductive Choice, an organization with ties to Planned Parenthood, began the Black Church Initiative to try to stop black churches from getting out of line. They choose the Reverend Carlton W. Veazey to head the group. Veazey makes Sharpton and Jackson look like Mother Theresa. He has stated

---

[139] Brian DeBose, "Black Churches Urged to Refocus," *Washington Times* 29 June 2006.

that abortion can be a "sacred choice."[140] When Veazey was questioned about Margaret Sanger's desire to exterminate the black race, he acknowledged that Sanger made unfortunate statements but that "charges of racism and genocide against Sanger are scare tactics."[141] He then added "the black community and religious leaders of our country would not be supporting us if we were pursing genocide."[142] This statement although seemingly intuitive is untrue, because those leaders could be ignorant of the plans or they could be scientific racist eugenicists, like W. E. B. Du Bois, who believe that they come from "good stock" unlike the vast majority of their fellow blacks who they believe are "human weeds."

Most arguments in favor of abortion focus on freedom of choice. Many have made more practical utilitarian arguments in favor of abortion. They say abortion can reduce crime and lower the welfare rolls. This argument is designed to appeal to

---

[140] Connie Schultz, "Minister Argues Abortion Can Be a 'Sacred Choice,'" http://www.canada.com/reginaleaderpost/news/churches/story.html?id=1405 bcf2-dbec-470d-929c-eb9d97bb5f71, 2 February 2006.
[141] Sheryl Blunt, "Saving Black Babies," http://www.christianitytoday.com/global/printer.html?/ct/2003/002/11.21.ht ml, 10 January 2003.
[142] Ibid.

those who would never have an abortion, but who are not principally opposed to others having abortions. Polls show that pro-lifers are passionate and often single-issue voters, while the pro-choice crowd is more apathetic. So how do you put fire in the belly of the pro-choice movement? Tell them it will reduce the welfare rolls and crime. Studies are sponsored to compare the cost of abortion to the cost of welfare. A study quoted in *Newsweek* said that the State of California should pay for abortions for welfare mothers because costs could rise if they don't: "Researchers estimate that it would have cost $464 million to provide one year's care children in lieu of abortions last year, which cost the state $27 million."[143] Planned Parenthood estimates that "Michigan taxpayers may have to shoulder between $23 million and $63 million in additional state public assistance costs from births occurring in 1991 as a result of a ban on Medicaid funding of abortion."[144] The Alan Guttmacher Institute estimates that abortions saved the

---

[143] Susan Fraker, Susan Agrest, Pamela Ellis Simons, Lucy Howard, Michael Reese, and Janet Hick, "Abortion Under Attack," *Newsweek*, 5 June 1978.
[144] Michael Klitsch, "Abortion Funding Cutoff Will Likely Cost Michigan Far More Than It Saves," *Family Planning Perspectives* (May 1994)

taxpayers $200 million in welfare expenses in 1976.[145] This cold cost-benefit analysis line of thought was paraphrased very succinctly by Evelyn Eaton of San Francisco's Catholic Council for Life when she said, "What they're saying is that a dead baby is cheaper than a live one."[146] It is interesting to note that Planned Parenthood is not known for its frugalness when spending tax dollars, but, when it comes to a living black baby on welfare or a dead one not on the welfare rolls, it become a fiscal conservative bean counter.

A 1969 advertisement linked birth control measures to a reduction in crime: "How many people do you want in your country? Already the cities are packed with youngsters. Thousand of idle victims of discontent and drug addiction. You go out after dark at your peril. . . . Birth control is the answer. . . . The evermounting tidal wave of humanity challenges us to control it, or be submerged along with all our civilized values."

Even recently, researchers have claimed that abortion reduces crime. The *New York Times* best seller *Freakonomics*

---

[145] Drogin, *Margaret Sanger*, 37.
[146] Fraker, et. al., "Abortion Under Attack."

stated that legal abortion reduces crime. Pro-lifer William Bennett criticized the book, saying, "But I do know that it's true that if you wanted to reduce crime, you could—if that were your sole purpose, you could abort every black baby in this country, and your crime rate would go down. That would be an impossible, ridiculous, and morally reprehensible thing to do, but your crime rate would go down. So these far-out, these far-reaching, extensive extrapolations are, I think, tricky." The media and the liberal establishment called him a racist for pointing out the racism inherent in the hypothesis that abortion reduces crime. This is a common tactic of Planned Parenthood and the establishment; they accuse their opponents of the very crimes they themselves are guilty of. They call their opponents racists when they are the ones trying to exterminate the black race. They call their opponents Nazis when their organization and their founder have ties to the Nazis and Hitler. They cannot defend their positions logically and morally, so they appeal to people's emotions hoping they never take the time to get the facts.

Chapter 7: Population Control

As we have seen, the eugenicists use many front arguments to advance their agenda. They sell abortions and birth control as a freedom of choice issue, as a way to save taxpayer's money, or as a way to reduce crime. One of their oldest and favorite front arguments is that there are too many people and the world's population must be reduced for the future of the planet. They call this argument "population control." Population control is not a new idea; it's a rehashed idea that was most famously promulgated by an eighteenth-century English intellectual Thomas Malthus in his now-discredited book *An Essay on the Principle of Population*. Malthus theorized that population grows at a faster rate than food supplies. He famously predicted that if the population were left unchecked, there would be massive famines in the middle of the nineteenth century. Of course, the exact opposite happened;

population grew and the people prospered because of productivity gains from the Industrial Revolution.

Malthus viewed the poor as a grave threat to civilization and thought people should abstain from giving charity to the poor. He advocated that poor people should be crowded together in order to "court the return of the plague" and that villages should be built "near stagnant pools"[147] to foster more diseases. He was also against teaching the poor healthy habits. He thought instead of "recommending cleanliness to the poor, we should encourage contrary habits."[148] Margaret Sanger's writings show Malthusian influences. In the following passage she claims that charity is worse than profiteering:

> The most serious charge that can be brought against modern 'benevolence'' is that it encourages the perpetuation of defectives, delinquents and dependents. These are the most dangerous elements in the world community, the most devastating curse on human progress and expression. Philanthropy is a gesture

---

[147] Grant, *Grand Illusions*, 26.
[148] Ibid., 33.

characteristic of modern business lavishing upon the unfit the profits extorted from the community at large. Looked at impartially, this compensatory generosity is in its final effect probably more dangerous, more dysgenic, more blighting than the initial practice of profiteering and the social injustice which makes some too rich and others too poor.[149]

All the evidence shows that all claims that there are too many people in the world are unequivocally false. If too many people were a cause of poverty, we would expect the most crowded countries to be the poorest and the least populated countries to be the richest. The data shows the exact opposite. Some of the most densely populated countries like Japan and Singapore are some of the richest countries, while some of the least populated countries like Nepal and Burma are some of the poorest nations.[150] A few hundred years ago many people suffered from hunger. Now because of technological advances

---

[149] Sanger, *The Pivot of Civilization*, 67.
[150] Jacqueline R. Kasun, *The War Against Population: The Economics and Ideology of World Population* (Ignatius Press, 1988), 52.

and freer economic systems, only 2 percent of the world's population suffers from serious hunger, and this hunger is a result of anti-free market government policies.[151] We are not running out of space either; less than half of the world's arable land is actually being farmed, and three-fourths of farmland needs no irrigation.[152] Even an official U.S. State Department study had to conclude "the economic case against rapid population growth . . . [is] . . . seriously flawed."[153]

There is much more evidence that is beyond the scope of this book. No serious economist gives any credence to the neo-Malthusian claims. Despite the overwhelming evidence that population growth does not cause poverty, the elites are engaged in a tax-dollar-financed plan to eradicate much of the world's population. The establishments of both political parties have shown that there are committed to population control.

During the Lyndon Johnson administration, in 1964, Congress passed the Economic Opportunity Act, and for the

---

[151] Ibid., 34.
[152] Ibid.
[153] Ibid., 50.

first time the federal government starting funding birth control.

Lyndon Johnson was a strong proponent of population control

measures. According to Security of State Dean Rusk and

National Security Adviser Walt Rostow, Johnson refused to

ship emergency wheat supplies to India during a famine in 1966

until that nation agreed to adopt a wide-scale birth control

program.[154] In 1968 Congress established the Center for

Population Research to manage the government's policies in

"population-related matters."[155] This bill even provided funding

for abortion research, placement, and services.[156]

    After the cultural revolution of the 1960s, the

establishment stepped up their rhetoric and increased funding of

eugenic policies disguised as population control measures. The

Richard Nixon and Jimmy Carter administrations were the most

openly eugenic administrations in the post-Holocaust era. In

1969 Nixon issued a "Special Message to the Congress on

Problems of Population Growth," calling for more federal

---

[154] Ibid., 86.
[155] Grant, *Grand Illusions*, 143.
[156] Ibid.,

funding for "family planning." Family planning was the new euphemistic term for birth control. In 1970 the Tydings Act increased funding for family planning. In 1974 the National Security Council completed a study called *Implications of Worldwide Population Growth for U.S. Security and Overseas Interests* (NSSM 20) that called the growing population in the third world as a threat to our national security and that measures should be taken to reduce their populations.[157] The surprisingly blunt memo even describes the cover story to be used to assuage any concerns that the native populations might have about population control:

> The U.S. can help to minimize charges of an imperialist motivation behind its support of population activities by repeatedly asserting that such support derives from a concern with:
>
> (a) the right of the individual couple to determine freely and responsibly their number and spacing of children

---

[157] Seamus Grimes, "The Ideology of Population Control in the UN Draft Plan for Cairo," *Population Research and Policy Review* 13, no. 3 (September 1994), 213.

and to have information, education, and the means to do

so; and

(b) the fundamental social and economic development of

poor countries in which rapid population growth is both

a contributing cause and a consequence of widespread

poverty.[158]

As amazing as this seems, the Orwellian "We are killing you for

your own good" or "It's all about choice and freedom" lines,

actually work. People are ignorant or refuse to believe that the

elites are engaged in an organized plot to kill most of the human

race. Of course it is not about choice and freedom. They

wouldn't be happy if every family in the third world *freely*

choose to have ten kids. In 1974 Robert McNamara, former

secretary of defense and president of the World Bank, went, as

far as to say that only thermonuclear war is a greater threat to

the world than population growth.[159]

---

[158] National Security Study Memorandum 200
[159] Stephen D. Mumford, "Abortion: A National Security Issue," *The Humanist* (September/October 1982)

Jimmy Carter continued the population control rhetoric and measures of Nixon. The Carter administration published *The Global 2000 Report to the President* that predicted "serious stresses" to natural resources by the year 2000, even though the same report admitted that the prices for natural resources have been declining. [160] Every first-year economic student knows that if the price of commodity is decreasing, that means one of three things: either demand is decreasing, supply is increasing, or both. Declining prices would not leave anybody with the slightest amount of knowledge of economics to predict shortages. In 1978, President Carter signed the Population Education Act authorizing federal funds to teach our children that there are too many people. Population control propaganda would be taught in "a broad array of subject fields such as geography, history, science, biology, social studies, and home economics."[161] A traveling exhibit was sent across the country with a frightening script that told children "We are running out of food. . . . we are running out of time." [162] The message to the

---

[160] Kasun, *The War Against Population,* 40
[161] Ibid., 166.

children was clear and stark. If more people don't die or if families don't start having fewer children, we will see massive starvation. Jimmy Carter warned of impending doom in his farewell address, "the *demands of increasing billions of people*, all combine to create problems which are easy to observe and predict but difficult to resolve. If we do not act, the world of *the year 2000 will be much less able to sustain life than it is now.* [emphasis mine]"

The farewell address of presidents traditionally have been used as a platform for presidents to tell the American people what they feel is the most pressing issue currently facing the country. George Washington used that moment to warn the people of the danger of "entangling alliances" with foreign nations and the importance of a noninterventionist foreign policy to stay out of unnecessary wars. Dwight Eisenhower warned the nation of the powerful military-industrial complex and its desire and ability to steer the republic into unnecessary wars. Those two men used the podium to try to save lives.

---

[162] Ibid., 21.

Jimmy Carter used his farewell address to spread more false eugenic population control nonsense in order to destroy life. The population control agenda continued under the Reagan, Bush I, Clinton, and George W. Bush administrations, and it continues today under Barack Obama. Barack Obama showed his commitment to eugenics with his first official act as president. Three days after his inauguration, Obama signed an executive order lifting a ban on using taxpayer dollars to fund abortions.[163] In the middle of the greatest financial crisis since the Great Depression, Obama's priority was not the financial concerns of the poor and the middle class, but was to make sure that tax dollars would fund abortions.

As much as the American establishment is dedicated to population control, it can't hold a candle to China. No country has launched a more successful eugenics campaign on its people under the banner of population control than China has. Like Hitler, the Chinese are the envy of the Western elites and have

---

[163] Jeff Mason and Deborah Charles, "Obama Lifts Restrictions on Abortion Funding,"
http://www.reuters.com/article/newsOne/idUSTRE50M3PQ20090123, 23 January 2009.

won their praises. If you want to see what kind of world we would live in if the elites had their druthers, look to China.

In China, students are expelled from schools if they get married, factory managers are told by the government how many children their employees can have, and family planning workers conduct brainwashing sessions to persuade people not to have children. If the brainwashing doesn't work, the government forces pregnant pheasant women to have an abortion if they have too many children.

"A reporter from Zhengming who visited eastern Guangdong reported how vigilantes abducted pregnant women on the streets and hauled them off, sometimes handcuffed or trussed, to abortion clinics. Other women, he said, were locked in detention cells or hauled before mass rallies and harangued into consenting to abortions. The reporter referred to 'aborted babies which were actually crying when they were born.'"[164]

Shockingly, a May 15, 1982, article in the *New York Times* tried to defend China's genocidal population controls as

---

[164] Christopher S. Wren, "China Birth Control Meet Regional Resistance," *New York Times*, 15 May 1982.

necessary, because "an expanding population is the biggest obstacle that China confronts in its push to modernize itself." The article neglects to mention that the most likely cause of Chinese poverty was China's centrally planned communist economy. In 1985 Taiwan was more than four times as crowded as mainland China, yet because the Taiwanese at the time had a relatively free economy, they had per capita income levels 8.5 times higher than the Chinese.[165] Another country with a free economy, the United Kingdom, was more than twice as crowded as China in 1985, yet they had income levels twenty-seven times that of the Chinese.[166]

The Chinese did not come up with their population control policy by themselves, it was designed by American population control experts and financed by U.S. tax dollars.[167] In 1999 United Nations Population Fund representative Sven Burmester praised China as having the "the most successful

---

[165] Kasun, *The War against Population*, 85.
[166] Ibid., 85.
[167] Ibid., 90.

family planning policy in the history of mankind in terms of quantity and with that, China has done mankind a favour."[168]

When it comes to population control, both the Republican and Democratic parties are staunchly in favor it. When it comes to abortion, it appears, to the casual observer, that there is disagreement between the parties. Most people believe that the Democratic Party is pro-abortion and the Republican Party is pro-life. But this is an illusion. Both parties have and are advancing the eugenics agenda of birth control and abortion. In fact, the eugenics movement has made some of its greatest advancements under Republican administrations. Five of the seven judges who voted to make abortion legal in the *Roe v. Wade* case were appointed by Republicans. A Republican majority appointed court upheld the *Roe v. Wade* decision in 1992 in the *Planned Parenthood v. Casey* case. Conservative icon Ronald Reagan wrote a letter praising Roger Pearson, a former member of the Eugenics Society and still an open racist

---

[168] Steven Mosher "Human Rights Triumphs over UNFPA Population Controllers" PRI Weekly Briefing http://www.lifeissues.net/writers/mos/mos_50humanrightswin.html, 17 June 2005.

and eugenicist, for his "substantial contributions to promoting and upholding those ideals and principles that we value at home and abroad."[169]

During the twelve years of the Reagan and the George H. W. Bush administrations, federal funding to Planned Parenthood tripled.[170] George W. Bush continued pro-abortion policies in the White House. The media myth that he is a Christian religious conservative gives him the perfect cover to advance the eugenics agenda. The media completely ignores his associations with occult organizations like Skull and Bones and the Bohemian Grove. When the South Dakota legislature passed a bill banning abortions in the state to challenge *Roe v. Wade,* Bush said he opposed the ban.[171] Bush also publicly stated that he would not ask his Supreme Court judge appointees if they would overturn *Roe v. Wade.* Bush also allowed the sale of the morning after pill, Plan B, which kills babies in the womb.[172]

---

[169] Kühl, *The Nazi Connection,* 4.

[170] Grant, *Grand Illusions*, 142.

[171] "Bush Disagrees with South Dakota Abortion Ban," *Agence France Presse*, 28 Feb 2006.

[172] "Bush Indicates Support for Plan B" *UPI* http://www.upi.com/Top_News/2006/08/21/Bush-indicates-support-for-Plan-B/UPI-86131156173565/, 21 August 2006.

The most common excuse by the Republicans is that we can't do anything about abortion because it is up to the Supreme Court. Even if you ignore the fact that most of the judges were appointed by Republicans, this is a pathetic and ridiculous excuse. One of the greatest myths perpetuated on the American public is that the Supreme Court has the power to overturn laws. This power does not exist in the Constitution. In fact the Founding Fathers warned about a too-powerful judicial branch. Thomas Jefferson stated, "It is a very dangerous doctrine to consider the judges as the ultimate arbiters of all constitutional questions; it is one which would place us under the despotism of an oligarchy." Abraham Lincoln also warned of an unelected court with the power to legislate. "The candid citizen must confess that if the policy of the government, upon vital questions, affecting the whole people, is to be irrevocably fixed by decisions of the Supreme Court . . . the people will have ceased to be their own rulers, having, to that extent, practically resigned their government into the hands of that eminent tribunal." Article III, Section II, of the Constitution gives the congress the power to say what is in the jurisdiction of the Supreme Court and what is not.

For six years, between 2000 and 2006, we had a Republican-controlled Senate, House, and White House. If the Republicans were truly against abortion, why didn't they pass a law stating the Supreme Court has no jurisdiction over abortion? The House used this power in the Marriage Protection Act. The Marriage Protection Act denied the Supreme Court any jurisdiction on the question of homosexual marriage by denying "all federal courts, including the Supreme Court, jurisdiction to rule on the constitutionality of the Defense of Marriage Act."[173] The reason they don't try to pass a similar law on abortion is that the Republican establishment, like the Democratic establishment, is in favor of eugenics.

The Bush family has historical ties to the eugenics movement, George W. Bush's grandfather, Prescott Bush, served as Connecticut state treasurer of Planned Parenthood.[174]

---

[173] Patrick J. Buchanan, "Has the Counterrevolution Begun?" http://www.lewrockwell.com/buchanan/buchanan8.html, 28 July 2004.
[174] Sidney Blumenthal, "Joe's Fall from Grace," http://www.salon.com/opinion/blumenthal/2006/08/09/lieberman_lamont/, 9 August 2006.

Prescott also provided funds for the Nazis during World War II, and the assets of the bank he ran, the Union Banking Corporation, were seized after the war by the federal government under the Trading with the Enemies Act.[175] As a congressman George H. W. Bush asked two "race-science" professors, William Shockley and Arthur Jensen, to testify before the Republican Task Force on Earth Resources and Population.[176] Some of William Shockley beliefs were a concern that "our nobly intended welfare programs may be encouraging dysgenics" and that "if those blacks with the least amount of Caucasian genes are in fact the most prolific and the least intelligent, then genetic enslavement will be the destiny of their next generation."[177] As a congressman, George H. W. Bush declared that he supported Planned Parenthood's goals 1,000 percent and compared population growth to a deadly virus like polio.[178]

---

[175] John Buchanan, "Bush—Nazi Link Confirmed," *New Hampshire Gazette*, http://www.nhgazette.com/articles/NN_Bush_Nazi_Link.html, 10 October 2003.
[176] Webster Griffin Tarpley and Anton Chaitkin, *George Bush: The Unauthorized Biography* (Progressive Press, 2006), 52.
[177] Ibid., 200.
[178] Ibid., 193, 195

Both the Republicans and the Democrats can't be trusted. They both are advancing the eugenics agenda. Their actions speak louder than words. The phony public abortion debate between the parties is just an elaborate good cop, bad cop, routine to squash any effective opposition to abortion, family planning, and eugenics. The passage quoted below is how Webster G. Tarpley and Anton Chaitkin in their biography of George H. W. Bush, *George Bush: The Unauthorized Biography*, describe the mind-set of George H. W. Bush. Although the authors were specifically writing about Bush, it could be applied to both the ruling elite on the left and the right:

One of our basic theses is that George Bush is, and considers himself to be, an oligarch. The notion of oligarchy includes first of all the idea of a patrician and wealthy family capable of introducing its offspring into such elite institutions as Andover, Yale, and Skull and Bones. Oligarchy also subsumes the self-conception of the oligarch as belonging to a special, exalted breed of mankind, one that is superior to the common run of mankind as a matter of hereditary genetic superiority. This mentality generally goes together with a fascination for eugenics, race science and just plain racism as a means of building a case that one's own family tree and racial stock are indeed superior. These notions of "breeding" are a constant in the history of the titled feudal aristocracy of Europe, especially Britain, towards inclusion in which an individual like Bush must necessarily strive. At the very least, oligarchs like Bush see themselves as demigods occupying a middle ground between the immortals above and the hoi polloi below. The culmination of this insane delusion, which Bush has demonstrably long since attained, is the obsessive belief that the principal families of the Anglo-American elite, assembled in their freemasonic orders, by themselves directly constitute an Olympian Pantheon of living deities who have the capability of abrogating and disregarding the laws of the universe according to their own irrational caprice."[179]

All the presidents since Lyndon Johnson have firmly been in Planned Parenthood's and the eugenicists' pocket, but probably none is better situated to advance Planned Parenthood's genocidal campaign against the black race than Barack Obama is. His black skin and African name make him the perfect Judas goat to lead blacks to the slaughterhouse. I personally witnessed a spontaneous celebration by blacks in Harlem on the night of his election. People were literally dancing in the streets and shouting his name. It was clear to me that the celebration had nothing to do with the man or his policies; it was an outburst of primitive tribalism. Barack Obama has become of symbol of black America. He has come to represent black America. With his victory, blacks felt they had won something. Because Obama is a symbol of black America, blacks will probably view any criticisms of him as personal criticisms and will reflexively defend him. His support

---

[179] Ibid., 9, 10

in black America is not based on logic and facts, but it is based on mob psychology and group think, and there is probably nothing Obama can do that will change black people's minds. Just like some sports fans that never believe the umpires make a bad call in their team's favor, blacks will never think any criticisms of Obama are justified.

Black people think they have won with the election of Obama. Let us look at what they have won. One thing they have won is a multibillion-dollar bailout of Wall Street bankers. Obama said that he would give money to people behind on their mortgages. Not one cent went to help people with their mortgages. Every dime went to the banks. Obama promised he would not raise taxes on families that make less than $250,000 and individuals that make less than $125,000. He lied. He pushed through Congress the "American Clean Energy and Security Act," otherwise known as the Cap and Trade bill, that will, by the government's own estimates, increase energy costs by the 19 percent.[180] This is a regressive tax, because it hits the poor the most. According to the Congressional Budget Office, the poor and the middle class will "see their paychecks cut between $880 and $1,500, or 2.9% to 2.7% of income," but the rich would only see a cut of 1.7 percent.[181] Obama promised during his campaign that all bills would be posted online for five days before they were voted on. He lied. The House of Representatives was not given the 1,200-page bill until 3:00 AM on the day of the vote. Of course, the bill still passed Congress anyway. During Obama's campaign, I never knew what his mindless empty campaign slogans, like "Yes we can" and "Change we can believe in," really meant. Apparently for Obama, "Yes we can" meant "Yes we can raise taxes on the poor and bailout the bankers."

I could list all of Obama's broken promises, but that would take another book and would probably still not convince Obama's brainwashed supporters. Obama is not just a tool of Wall Street; he also has close ties to Planned Parenthood.

---

[180] Robert Schroeder, "Climate Bill Would Lead to Increased Costs, Study Says," http://www.marketwatch.com/story/climate-bill-would-lead-to-increased-costs-study-2009-08-04, 4 August 2009.
[181] "Who Pays for Cap and Trade?" http://online.wsj.com/article/SB123655590609066021.html, 9 March 2009.

Planned Parenthood president Cecile Richards bragged after meeting at the White House on her twitter page that, "Just left the White House meeting on women's health care—they appreciate all the mighty PP supporters speaking up for reform in the states!"[182] Obama's health-care plan has money for Planned Parenthood to provide for "reproductive health." "Reproductive health" is an umbrella term the eugenicists use for birth control and abortion. When pressed by Katie Couric whether his health care plan would cover abortions, he was evasive and dodged the question: "What I think is important, at this stage, is not trying to micromanage what benefits are covered. Because I think we're still trying to get a framework. And my main focus is making sure that people have the options of high quality care at the lowest possible price."[183]

Obama wasn't so evasive about using tax dollars to fund abortions in Washington, D.C. Washington, D.C., has a

---

[182] Kathleen Gilbert, "Planned Parenthood Continues Boasting Close Ties with White House on Obamacare Bill," http://www.lifesitenews.com/ldn/2009/aug/09081403.html, 14 August 2009.
[183] Kathleen Gilbert, "Obama: 'Let's Not Get Distracted' over Taxpayer-Funded Abortion Coverage in Healthcare," http://www.lifesitenews.com/ldn/2009/jul/09072212.html, 22 July 2009.

majority black population, so it should be no surprise that Obama's budget recommendations called for tax dollars to be used to fund abortions in the Washington, D.C.[184] Obama may be the most proabortion politician on the national stage. He has made it clear that abortion is one of his top priorities. He told Planned Parenthood that, "The first thing I'd do as president is sign the Freedom of Choice Act." The Freedom of Choice Act would strike down every state law restricting abortion, including parental notification laws. Obama is so in favor of abortion that in 2001 he was the only Illinois senator to speak against a bill that would ban the killing of babies that survived an abortion and were living outside the womb.[185]

When he is not advocating taxpayer-funded abortion on demand, he is pushing for sex education for five year olds. When criticized during an Illinois senate debate for supporting sex education for Kindergartners, Obama responded, "But it's the right thing to do, to provide age-appropriate sex education,

[184] Kathleen Gilbert, "Obama White House Urges Tax-Funded Abortion-on-Demand in D.C.,"
http://www.lifesitenews.com/ldn/2009/may/09050812.html, 8 May 2009.
[185] Jerome R. Corsi, *The Obama Nation*:Threshold Editions, 2008), 238.

science-based sex education in schools."[186] His 2010 budget calls for $150 million in condom based education.[187] He also has praised Planned Parenthood's National Black Church Initiative, saying, "We need more programs in our communities like the National Black Church Initiative, which empowers our young people by teaching them about reproductive health, sex education."[188]

From the beginning of the birth control, or family planning, movement there have been black leaders who have spoken against it. In 1934, at the annual convention of Marcus Garvey's Universal Negro Improvement Association, a resolution condemning birth control was passed unanimously.[189] It warned blacks not to "accept or practice the theory of birth control such as is being advocated by irresponsible speculators who are attempting to interfere with the course of nature and with the

---

[186] Tahman Bradley, "Obama Targeted on 'Sex Ed for Kindergarteners," http://blogs.abcnews.com/politicalradar/2008/09/obama-targeted.html, 9 September 2008.
[187] Kathleen Gilbert, "Obama Calls for Condom Funding to Replace Abstinence Education," http://www.lifesitenews.com/ldn/2009/may/09051203.html, 12 May 2009.
[188] Corsi, *The Obama Nation*, 239.
[189] Weisbord, *Genocide?*, 43.

purpose of the God in whom we believe."[190] Elijah Muhammad, leader of the Nation of Islam, cautioned blacks of not "being trapped into the kind of disgraceful birth control laws now aimed exclusively at poor, helpless black peoples who have no one to rely on."[191] After the Nation of Islam's newspaper, *Muhammad Speaks*, ran a series attacking the birth control movement, Planned Parenthood sent representatives to Malcolm X in an attempt to persuade him that there were no evil intentions behind the movement. Malcolm X, to his credit, was unconvinced and refused to change his anti-birth control position.[192] Blacks in Cleveland took matters in their own hands and burned a birth control clinic when they saw through the machinations of the birth control and family planning propaganda and figured out it was a plan for genocide.[193] Erma Craven, a black pioneer in the pro-life movement, made the observation, "In time past, the Blacks couldn't grow kids fast enough for their 'masters' to harvest; now that power is near,

---

[190] Ibid.
[191] Ibid., 98.
[192] Ibid., 98–99.
[193] John Sibley, "'Wanted' Babies Said to Cause U.S. Population Expansion," *New York Times*, 15 November 1968.

the masters want us to call a moratorium on having babies. When looked at in context, the whole mess adds up to blatant genocide."[194]

Blacks have not only spoken out but have also taken action. A coalition of ministers, parents, and educators sued the Chicago Board of Education, charging that the city's school-based clinics were a form of discrimination and a violation of the state's fortification laws. Their suit stated that the clinics are "designed to control the Black population" and are "calculated, pernicious effort to destroy the very fabric of family life among Black parents and their children." Tanya Crawford, a parent involved in the suit, commented when she saw literature they handed her daughter in school, "I never realized how racist those people were until I read the things they were giving Dedrea at the school clinic. They're as bad as the Klan. Maybe worse, because they're so slick and sophisticated. Their bigotry is all dolled up with statistics and surveys, but just beneath the

---

[194] D. L. Cuddy, "Black Genocide," *America* (3 October 1981): 181.

surface it's as ugly as apartheid. It's as ugly as anything I can imagine.[195]

Today, the number of blacks trying to warn blacks about the true nature of family planning is only increasing. LEARN INC. (Life Education And Resource Network) is one of those organizations; it describes itself as the "largest, African-American, evangelical pro-life ministry in the United States." Its Web site, http://learninc.org/, contains many articles exposing the true goals of family planning and the proabortion movement. Pastor Clenard Howard Childress Jr. is the leader of the northeast chapter of LEARN. He is an outspoken and effective spokesman and is frequently quoted and featured in the Christian press. His Web site, http://www.blackgenocide.org, is an excellent resource for those wanting to learn more about this issue

Chapter 8: AIDS

---

[195] Grant, *Grand Illusions*, 109–10.

For the most part, the eugenicists prefer soft kill methods of extermination, like birth control, abortion, and sterilization. These methods are considered soft kill rather than fast kill, because they are less direct and reduce the size of the population slowly. Fast kill methods, like Hitler's gas chamber, work faster, but the efficiency comes with a great cost because it is more likely to spark resistance from the target population. Here lies the great conundrum for the eugenicists. Every tactic that kills people at a fast rate is more likely to lead to backlash that could crush the eugenics movement once and for all. The eugenicists may have the perfect weapon to solve this conundrum. It works fast and it leaves no trail back to them. Race-specific bio weapons, deadly viruses designed in a laboratory to kill only specific races. No one would suspect that the virus was created in a lab and the deaths of millions of people would be looked upon only as unfortunate accident of nature that human beings are powerless to stop.

There is and has been a lot of interest in elite circles in the creation of race-specific diseases. The *Washington Post* reported that South Africa was working on race-specific biological weapons to kill the black population while leaving the white population unharmed.[196] The Israelis are working on a bioweapon that will kill Arabs but leave Jews unaffected.[197] The U.S. government has also launched similar investigations. A November 1970 article in the *Military Review*, the professional journal of the U.S. Army, speculates and describes how bioweapons targeting specific ethnic groups could be created and used.[198] In 2000 *The Project for a New American Century* (PNAC), a think tank with government ties and widely considered to be the intellectual architects of the War on Terror and the war in Iraq, wrote a paper that stated "advanced forms of biological warfare that can 'target' specific genotypes [races] may transform biological warfare from the realm of terror to a politically useful tool."[199] Members of PNAC include former

---

[196] Joby Warrick and John Mintz, "Lethal Legacy: Bioweapons for Sale; U.S. Declined South African Scientist's Offer on Man-Made Pathogens," *Washington Post*, 20 April 2003

[197] "Israel's Ethnic Weapon?" http://www.wired.com/news/politics/0,1283,16272,00.html, 16 November 1998.

[198] Carl A. Larsen, "Ethnic Weapons," *Military Review* (November 1970): 3–11.

[199] *The Project for a New American Century, Present Dangers: Crisis and Opportunity in American Foreign and Defense Policy.*

Secretary of Defense Donald Rumsfeld, Vice President Dick Cheney, Paul Wolfowitz, and Richard Perle. The World Health Organization (WHO) also funded and conducted research into the genetic disease vulnerabilities of Africans, American Indians, and other minority groups.[200]

A disease like AIDS is exactly the type of disease the eugenicists would want. For starters, it is a deadly disease. It also attacks the immune system, making it difficult for the human body to defend itself and develop immunity to the virus. A deadly virus that hits a group can make that group stronger because that group can develop immunity to the virus. One of the reasons the Europeans were able to conquer the indigenous people of North and South America is that they had immunity to diseases, like small pox, that the Native Americans had never before encountered. Because AIDS is transmitted through sexual intercourse, it discourages people from having sex without using condoms. This of course, has the added benefit of helping to lower the birthrate. Although AIDS has hit the white

---

[200] Leonard G. Horowitz, *Emerging Virus* (Tetrahedron, 1996), 12.

population, it has moved the fastest among the black population. Since the beginning of the AIDS epidemic, scientists have noticed that AIDS develops unusually slowly in some people and others get HIV, yet never contract AIDS. Scientific studies show that AIDS is a more deadly virus with nonwhites than with whites. Stephen O'Brien and Michael Dean published the results of a study in the September 1997 issue of the *Scientific America*, in an article entitled "In Search of AIDS-Resistance Genes," that found that certain people are born with AIDS-resistance genes. According to this study, the AIDS-resistant gene is mostly found among whites and rarely found in black Americans. "The HIV-resistance allele, or deletion mutant, of the CCR5 gene is not distributed equally among the world's peoples. It is virtually absent in African and eastern Asian populations and in Native Americans and is rare in African-Americans [see second column in table below]. It is, however, fairly prevalent among Caucasians (descendants of the early settlers of Europe and western Asia)."[201]

---

[201] Stephen J. O'Brien and Michael Dean, "In Search of AIDS-Resistance Genes," *Scientific American* 277, no. 3 (September 1997)

The statistics of AIDS infections certainly substantiate that AIDS has predilection toward the world's colored people. The region in the world hit hardest by AIDS is Sub-Sahara Africa. According to the United Nations, one-tenth of the world's population lives in Sub-Sahara Africa, but 64 percent of HIV cases are in that region.[202] Globally, the United Nations estimates the infection rate among adults to be 1 percent, and the only regions they estimate to have higher infection rate are the world's two primarily black regions; Sub-Saharan Africa at 6.1 percent and the Caribbean at 1.6 percent.[203] In the United States, the Centers for Disease Control (CDC) estimates that 47 percent of the AIDS cases in America were non-Hispanic blacks even though blacks only account for 13 percent of the population.[204] Things are only getting worse; blacks accounted for 51 percent of new AIDS diagnoses between 2001 and 2004.[205] If AIDS is man-made, it appears to be the perfect race specific

---

[202] "2006 Report on the global AIDS epidemic" United Nations, 15.
[203] Ibid., Annex 2: "HIV and AIDS Estimates and Data."
[204] "Racial/Ethnic Disparities in Diagnoses of HIV/AIDS—33 States, 2001–2004," *Morbidity and Mortality Weekly Report Centers for Disease Control and Prevention*, 55, no. 5, Centers for Disease Control and Prevention. Vol. 55 Issue No. 05, —.
[205] Ibid.

bio weapon. Is there any evidence that AIDS is man-made? To answer that, we should first ask, where did AIDS come from?

The theory popularized by the mainstream media is that AIDS comes from an African green monkey. Very succinctly, the green monkey theory is that some African was either bitten by, had sex with, or ate a monkey that gave him AIDS. AIDS spread from the monkey, to the African, to the rest of the world. The evidence shows that this story is not only false, but also completely ridiculous. AIDS sprang up simultaneously among white homosexuals in urban areas in the United States and among urban heterosexuals in Africa. First, if AIDS came from green monkeys, it would have infected rural Africans before urban Africans; yet the reverse is the case, AIDS was found among urban Africans before rural Africans. The pygmies live and eat the green monkeys, but they got AIDS after city-dwelling Africans got AIDS. Second, in America, AIDS originated with white homosexuals and was known for a time as a gay disease. But in Africa, AIDS originated in the heterosexual population. It seems inconceivable that AIDS would go from a green monkey in the bush to urban heterosexual Africans to white American homosexuals. Even if such a scenario was possible, it couldn't have happened, because AIDS sprang up among Africans and American homosexuals at the same time. Third, in 1988 University of Tokyo researchers found no genetic link between the AIDS-like virus found in the monkeys and the virus that is found in humans.[206] The link between AIDS and the African green monkey has been so thoroughly debunked that no one in the scientific community currently believes in it.

Many scientists and researchers have developed a more plausible alternate theory about the origin of the AIDS virus. Their research and examination of the evidence has led them to believe that AIDS is a man-made virus. One of the researchers who believes that AIDS is man-made is Dr. Robert Strecker, M.D., a medical consultant. Dr. Robert Strecker was hired by the Security Pacific Bank to research the impact of AIDS on the firm's health insurance policies. His research led him to believe

---

[206] Robert Steitnbrook, "Research Refutes Idea That Human AIDS Virus Originated in Monkeys," *Los Angeles Times*, 2 June 1988: p. 3.

that AIDS was man-made, and he produced a video, the *Strecker Memorandum*, documenting the evidence that led him to that conclusion. Dr. Alan Cantwell, M.D., a scientific researcher, has written two books, *AIDS and the Doctors of Death: An Inquiry into the Origin of the AIDS Epidemic* and *Queer Blood: The Secret AIDS Genocide Plot*, claiming that AIDS is an artificially created disease. Dr. Len Horowitz, M.D., a Harvard graduate and former Harvard faculty member, also believes AIDS was created in a government laboratory and has documented how he came to that conclusion in his book, *Emerging Viruses: AIDS And Ebola: Nature, Accident or Intentional?* Dr. John Seale, M.D., writing in the September 1988, Volume 81, British *Journal of the Royal Society of Medicine* noted that "The technology required to produce, artificially, epidemics of HIV-1, HIV-2 and other new retroviruses pathogenic to man was already available in the 1960s" and that "it is as plausible that the AIDS viruses were produced artificially as naturally."[207] Kenyan ecologist and

---

[207] John Seale, "Origins of the AIDS Viruses, HIV-1 and HIV-2: Fact or Fiction?" *British Journal of the Royal Society of Medicine* 81 (September

Nobel Peace Prize winner, Wangari Maathai, has stated her belief that AIDS was "created by a scientist for biological warfare."[208] German microbiologist Jacob Segal also believes that AIDS was man-made.[209]

Although much of the evidence that has led scientists to believe AIDS is man-made is scientific and beyond the scope of most laymen's understanding, there is other traditional, nonscientific evidence that points to a man-made origin of AIDS. Here are some facts that even the most strident skeptics of the man-made origin theory of AIDS cannot deny. First, the U.S. government and WHO spent money to research and develop an AIDS-like virus that attacks the immune system in the same manner as AIDS. Second, government scientists did develop an AIDS-like virus before AIDS became public and published their findings in scientific research journals. Third, there is evidence that the first AIDS patients were infected

---

1988): 537–39.

[208] Kenyan Wangari, "Nobel Peace Laureate Claims HIV Deliberately Created," http://www.abc.net.au/news/newsitems/200410/s1216687.htm, 9 October 2004.

[209] Alan Cantwell, *Aids and the Doctors of Death* (Aries Rising Press, 1988), 185.

through contaminated vaccinations they received while participating in mass vaccination programs administered and funded by the WHO and the U.S. government, the same organizations that allocated resources to develop a virus to attack the immune system.

On July 1, 1969, Dr. Donald M. MacArthur, a spokesman for the Department of Defense, appeared before the House Subcommittee of the Committee on Appropriations in Congress and made a request for $10 million to develop a virus. Dr. MacArthur stated that he wanted "to produce a synthetic biological agent, an agent that does not naturally exist and for which no natural immunity could have been acquired." MacArthur wanted the virus to be synthetic because all naturally occurring viruses "are known by scientists throughout the world" and it therefore makes it easier for scientists to develop cures. A synthetic virus, on the other hand, would not be well known and therefore it would be more difficult to develop a cure. Most important, he also wanted the virus to attack the immune system, thereby making it harder for the human body to fight the virus and develop immunity to the virus. It would be perfect virus, difficult, if not impossible, for both scientists and the human immune system to fight and defeat. MacArthur made a very persuasive argument, and Congress granted his request. Below is a transcript of Dr. MacArthur's testimony before Congress (emphasis mine):[210]

There are two things about the biological agent field I would like to mention. One is the possibility of technological surprise. Molecular biology is a field that is advancing very rapidly, and eminent biologists believe that within a period of 5 to 10 years it **would be possible to produce a synthetic biological agent, an agent that does not naturally exist and for which no natural immunity could have been acquired.**

Mr. Sikes. Are we doing any work in that field?

[210] Horowitz, *Emerging Virus*, 6–7.

Dr. MacArthur. We are not.

Mr. Sikes. Why not? Lack of money or lack of interest?

Dr. MacArthur. Certainly not lack of interest.

[MacArthur provides the following information:]

1. **All biological agents up to the present time are representatives of naturally occurring diseases, and thus are known by scientists throughout the world. They are easily available to qualified scientists for research, either for offensive or defensive purposes.**

2. Within the next 5 to 10 years, it would probably be possible to make a new infective microorganism which could differ in certain important aspects from any known disease-causing organisms. **Most important of these is that it might be refractory to the**

immunological and therapeutic processes upon which we depend to maintain our relative freedom from infectious disease.

3. A research program to explore the feasibility of this could be completed in approximately 5 years at a total cost of $10 million.

4. It would be very difficult to establish such a program. Molecular biology is a relatively new science. There are not many competent scientists in the field, almost all are in university laboratories, and they are generally adequately supported from sources other than the Department of Defense. However, it was considered possible to initiate an adequate program through the National Academy of Sciences—National Research Council (NAS-NRC). The matter was discussed with the NAS-NRC, and tentative plans were made to initiate the program. However, decreasing funds in CB

(chemical/biological) research, growing criticism of the CB program, and our reluctance to involve the NAS-NRC in such a controversial endeavor have led us to postpone it for the past two years. **It is a highly controversial issue and there are many who believe such research should not be undertaken lest it lead to yet another method of massive killing of large populations**. . . . Should an enemy develop it, there is little doubt that it is an important area of potential military technological inferiority in which there is no adequate research program.

It turns out that the Defense Department wasn't the only one interested in finding a virus to attack the immune system. The WHO, which receives the majority of its funding from the U.S. government, also expressed an interest in creating an AIDS-like virus that attacks the immune system. The 1972 WHO Bulletin recommends that "An attempt should be made to see if viruses can in fact exert selective effects on immune function. . . . The possibility should be looked into that the immune response to the virus itself may be impaired if the inflicting virus damages, more or less selectively, the cell responding to the virus."[211]

The World Health Organization is ostensibly an organization devoted to improving people's health and saving lives, so it seems rather strange that its leaders believe and voice the standard eugenics population growth propaganda. In May 1978, before the AIDS epidemic broke out, Joseph A. Califano, the United State's secretary of health, education, and welfare, led a delegation to the thirty-first assembly of the WHO. In his speech he claimed that population growth "retards social and economic progress in many nations and burdens families and communities."[212] Again, anyone researching eugenics will be constantly amazed at the frankness and boldness of those in the eugenics movement to openly state their belief that there are too many people. After telling the assembly that there are too many people, Califano announced the United States' commitment to

---

[211] "Virus Associated Immunopathology: Animal Models and Implications for Human Disease," *WHO Bulletin* 47, no. 2 (1972): 259.
[212] Horowitz, *Emerging Virus*, 172.

"battle against infectious diseases" by vaccinating people in the third world and establishing a disease research center in Africa.[213] Why would he be interested reducing population and also be interested in improving health? These seem like contradictory goals. As we will see, the WHO is just another eugenics front organization and the vaccinations Califano proposed did not fight diseases but were contaminated and gave deadly diseases to the recipients. Instead of hiding under the banner of "personal liberties and privacy" like Planned Parenthood, the WHO hides under the banner of concern for the health of the poor.

We know that the U.S. government specifically requested for an "an agent that does not naturally exist and for which no natural immunity could have been acquired" to be created. We know that AIDS fits the characteristics of the virus the government requested. But do we have any evidence that such a virus was ever created by the U.S. government? In 1969 Dr. Robert Gallo, chief of the Laboratory of Tumor Cell Biology at the National Cancer Institute (NCI), and Robert

---

[213] Ibid., 173.

Ting, an employee of biological warfare defense contractor Litton Bionetics, published in a medical journal that they had modified a virus found in monkeys with cat leukemia to create cancers that are commonly seen in AIDS patients.[214] Gallo also presented papers to a NATO-sponsored symposium on ways to create an AIDS-like virus.[215] According to Dr. Leonard G. Horowitz, who studied Gallo and his colleagues' work published in scientific journals, Gallo and other government scientists had "created numerous AIDS-like viruses for more than a decade before" AIDS was officially discovered.[216]

The fact that Dr. Gallo worked on creating AIDS-like viruses before the AIDS epidemic with known defense contractors is not even the most incriminating evidence against him. The most incriminating evidence is his strange behavior after the AIDS epidemic began. When the AIDS epidemic began in 1980, scientists had still not isolated the virus and very little about the virus was known. Because little was known,

---

[214] Ibid., 70.
[215] Ibid.
[216] Ibid., 75.

scientists could not develop a vaccine for AIDS or even work on a blood test for the disease. Gallo, the NCI's lead expert on viruses, showed remarkably little interest in AIDS when the epidemic began. The NCI withheld funds for scientists who wanted to research AIDS. Gallo "withheld experimental reagents including the antibodies needed to identify AIDS-like viruses."[217] When Jim Mullins, a Harvard biologist, reported to the CDC his research on AIDS, Gallo scolded him publicly for forty-five minutes, accusing him of being an ingrate and for going behind his back. Mullins believed that Gallo was angry because he felt Mullins might have found the virus, "Gallo thought I may have found the virus."[218]

Gallo appeared to have almost no interest in AIDS until April of 1983, when Luc Montagnier of the world-renowned Pasteur Institute in France appeared to have isolated the AIDS virus. Montagnier sent a sample of the virus taken from a Frenchman with AIDS-like symptoms to Gallo for him to study.

---

[217] Ibid., 57.
[218] Seth Roberts, "What AIDS Researcher Dr. Robert Gallo Did in Pursuit of the Nobel Prize," *Spy Magazine* (July 1990)

Montagnier thought that this might be the AIDS virus, and he published his findings in the May 1983 issue of the *Science* journal. The scientific community largely overlooked Montagnier's findings, choosing to wait until Gallo passed his judgment. Gallo never passed judgment. Instead on April 23, 1984, Margaret Heckler, secretary of health and human services, announced that Robert Gallo had discovered the AIDS virus and that a blood test would be soon available and a vaccine would be two years away.

The problem was that Gallo's virus was the exact same virus that the French had isolated before and sent to Gallo to review. Gallo just renamed the virus and said he discovered it. Gallo wanted all the credit and the money that would come with a patent on the blood test. Eventually, the French and Gallo came to a settlement and agreed to split credit and all revenues from the blood test. Gallo's behavior is rather schizophrenic; he went from being completely disinterested in the AIDS virus to being a reckless ego maniac willing to risk his reputation to establish himself as the founder of the AIDS virus.

His behavior does make sense if he was the creator of the AIDS virus. If he created the virus, his first instinct would be to use his position and high standing to stonewall any attempts to fight the virus. But when it came apparent that the virus would be found, he would want to make sure he would be credited with finding it. Now Gallo is now credited as the cofounder of the AIDS virus, and that status gives him tremendous power to influence the direction of AIDS research. If he was the creator of the AIDS virus, he could use that power to thwart efforts to find a cure or the true cause of the disease. Gallo is also the creator and main propagator of the claim that AIDS originated from the green monkey myth. Because he is known as the cofounder of the AIDS virus, the media has given tremendous credibility to his theories on the true origin of AIDS and he is able to divert any attention to the man made origin theory of AIDS.

If AIDS is a man-made disease, the most difficult task is not creating the disease but infecting the victims with the disease. Most people are not going to just allow a stranger stick a needle in their arm. What if you could trick your victims into allowing you to stick a needle in them? The evidence suggests that the eugenicists did just that. By using a cover story that the needles were vaccinations that would protect people from disease, they were able to infect unsuspecting victims with the AIDS virus. History has repeatedly shown the maxim never trust your enemies when they are bearing gifts to be wise advice. In the midst of the French and Indian war, the British commander in chief, Sir Jeffrey Amherst, was outnumbered by Indians and was concerned that the Indians would defeat his troops at Fort Pitt. He devised a plan and wrote to one of his captains that smallpox should be spread among the Indian tribes with contaminated blankets. "You will do well to try to inoculate the Indians by means of blankets as well as to try every other method that can serve to extirpate this exorable race."[219] In June of 1763, Captain Ecuyer met with two Indian chiefs and, as a token of friendship, offered them blankets that had been taken from the smallpox hospital. Captain Ecuyer's

---

[219] Leonard A. Cole *Clouds of Secrecy: The Army's Germ Warfare Tests over Populated Areas* : Littlefield Adams Quality Paperbacks, 1988, 12.

gift led to a smallpox epidemic among the tribes in the area. The eugenicists' tactics are very similar to Captain Ecuyers'; they always seek to make their victims unwittingly accomplices in their own destruction.

A May 11, 1987, *London Times* article entitled "Smallpox Vaccine 'Triggered Aids Virus'" offered another hypothesis on the origin of AIDS virus. The article noted that the outbreak of AIDS in Africa coincided with a massive wide-scale smallpox vaccination program performed by the United Nation's WHO: "The greatest spread of HIV infection coincides with the most intense immunization programmes, with the number of people immunised being as follows: Zaire 36,878,000; Zambia 19,060,000; Tanzania 14,972,000; Uganda 11,616,000; Malawai 8,118,000; Ruanda 3,382,000 and Burundi 3,274,000. Brazil, the only South American country covered in the eradication campaign, has the highest incidence of Aids in that region. About 14,000 Haitians, on United Nations secondment to Central Africa, were covered in the campaign."[220]

A WHO adviser looked at the evidence and stated, "I thought it was just a coincidence until we studied the latest findings about the reactions which can be caused by Vaccinia. Now I believe the smallpox vaccine theory is the explanation to the explosion of aids."[221] This story appeared all over the European press, but no major American news organization covered the story. Could this have been a coincidence? Could it be that the people who contracted AIDS just so happened to be the same people who received the vaccination? This sounds like a highly improbable scenario. Even stranger is that the same scenario took place in the United States at the same time; the first cases of AIDS in America just happened to be found in a group that also took part in a vaccination program.

Around the same time AIDS was erupting in Africa, AIDS began to affect white homosexuals in the United States. Just before AIDS broke out in the United States, Wolf Szmuness, a defector from the Soviet Union, was given the

---

[220] Pearce Wright, "Smallpox Vaccine 'Triggered AIDS Virus,'" *London Times*, 11 May 1987.
[221] Ibid.

important job of managing an experimental Hepatitis-B vaccine experiment. The experiment was sponsored by the Centers for Disease Control, the National Institute of Health, the National Institute of Allergy and Infectious Diseases, Abbott Laboratories, and Merck, Sharp & Dohme. Szmuness did not use any heterosexual men for the experiment. He insisted on using promiscuous, professional, primarily white, homosexual men. The first study took place in New York City, and just after the study AIDS broke out in New York City's homosexual community. Similar experiments were later conducted with homosexual white men in San Francisco, Los Angeles, Denver, St. Louis, and Chicago. AIDS epidemics broke out in those cities among homosexual men shortly after the tests were conducted. When the blood of the men who participated in the New York experiment was tested in 1985, it showed that 20 percent of the men tested positive for HIV in 1980. No place in the world and no sample, including in Africa, ever recorded a higher infection rate of HIV in 1980.

Researchers only had the opportunity to test the blood, because Szmuness had requested that all 13,000 vials of blood from the men in the experiment be stored. This was an unusual request because of the cost and space needed to store that much blood, but Szmuness insisted, stating, "Because one day another disease may erupt and we'll need this material."[222] That is a rather odd comment from somebody running a vaccination program. Szmuness must have suspected that the vaccination program had an ulterior purpose and that the vaccinations were contaminated. Szmuness' suspicions make more sense when put into the context of his life.

Szmuness had a hard life. He was a Jew and originally from Poland. He lost his family in the German concentration camps, and he fled to the Soviet Union to escape from the Germans. The Soviets sent him to a work camp in Siberia. Szmuness' frail body was not suited for the hard labor and he soon grew ill from malnutrition and the excruciating Russian winters. The Russians, realizing that he could die and he would

[222] June Goodfield, *Quest for the Killers:* Birkhäuser, 1985, 92.

be no use dead, wisely decided to reassign the doctor and placed him in charge of controlling outbreaks of lice and other infectious diseases. The Russians also wanted to use the doctor as a spy on internal enemies. Szmuness initially refused to spy for the KGB, but he relented and agreed to be a spy after intensive psychological and physical torture. His KGB tormentors told him, "Say nothing of this to anyone, but remember. We will reach you anywhere in the world. No matter where you go, no matter where you try to hide, you will never be out of our grasp."[223] After the war the Russians allowed him to return his native Poland, then under communist control. In Poland he became a celebrity for discovering the cause of an epidemic of enteric fever. His popularity with the communists soon faded when he refused to publicly criticize Israel during the Six Days' War. Because of his refusal, he was fired from his job. According to the official story, faced with no job, dwindling savings, and a family to feed, he defected with his wife and children to the United States in 1969.

---

[223] Ibid., 57.

There are some red flags in the official Szmuness story. First, he defected when the Soviets allowed him and his family to attend a conference in Italy. It was standard practice for the Soviets to keep the family of anyone allowed to leave the country in the Soviet Union as a deterrent against defection. Why would they make an exception with a valuable asset like Szmuness? Szmuness was one of the world's leading experts in hepatitis and an informant for the KGB. Surely the communists would not want to lose someone so valuable to the Americans, and they would take the normal precautions to ensure against his defection. When he arrived in America, the FBI did not question him to ascertain if he was a double agent. There were no articles in the newspapers, gloating over the defection of a leading scientist of the hated Soviets to the United States. He was just quietly given a job at the New York Blood Center, and within five years a new department was created specifically for him to run. His story gets stranger. When Szmuness returned to the Soviet Union in 1975, he experienced no repercussions from the Soviet government but was welcomed back as a hero.

Needless to say, this was not how the Soviets usually treated those who defected. Despite the cold war, Americans and the Russians did share secrets about biological warfare.[224] Was Szmuness lent to the Americans as part of joint biological warfare research program? Szmuness may have agreed to this, in exchange for being allowed to flee the Soviet Union with his family. Was his insisting that vials of blood be stored an act of defiance against his captors?

We may never know the answers to those questions, but the AIDS vaccination program is not an isolated incident; the WHO and the U.S. government have been caught many times giving people contaminated vaccinations. In 1995 in the Philippines the WHO launched an ambitious tetanus vaccination program targeting women of childbearing age (fifteen to forty-five). The fact that only childbearing women were given the vaccine raised eyebrows because tetanus is a disease that attacks both sexes. Suspicions were further aroused when many pregnant women had spontaneous abortions when given the

---

[224] Horowitz, *Emerging Virus*, 24–25, 28–29.

vaccine. Because of pressure from concerned citizens, the Philippine Department of Health tested the vaccine and found that 20 percent of the sample tested positive for the hormone human chorionic gonadotrophin (hCG). hCG is a known anti-pregnancy agent that causes spontaneous abortions in pregnant women and renders women infertile. This is not the only case of the WHO vaccinating people in a third world with vaccines contaminated with anti-pregnancy agents. The Nigerian government caught UNICEF and the WHO injecting people with a polio vaccine contaminated with hCG in 2004.[225]

The U.S. government has admitted that from 1955 to 1963 American children were vaccinated with a Polio vaccine contaminated with a cancer-causing virus called SV40. Even though the Department of Health was aware of the contamination in 1961, they continued to use it for two more years. Cancers linked to the SV40 virus are more common than in the past; the incidences of ependymoma is up 25 percent,

---

[225] "UNICEF Nigerian Polio Vaccine Contaminated with Sterilizing Agents Scientist Finds—Scientist Says Things Discovered in Vaccines Are 'Harmful, Toxic,'" http://www.lifesite.net/ldn/2004/mar/04031101.html, 11 March 2004.

bone malignancies are up 23 percent, and mesothelioma is up 90 percent. The Baylor College of Medicine found that 40 percent of non-Hodgkin lymphomas tumors contained the exact strain of SV40 found in the polio vaccines.[226]

The AIDS epidemic erupted at the same time among two disparate groups that couldn't be more different from each other: white professional urban American gays and heterosexual Africans. Not only are these two groups separated by a thousand miles and an ocean, but there are of different races, cultures, nationalities, socioeconomic classes, and sexual preferences. How could AIDS have possibly begun with these two groups at the same time? This could not have incurred naturally. The only connection is that both groups participated in vaccination programs. It stretches logic and the laws of probability to believe that two disparate demographic groups separated by an ocean, race, and many other factors were infected at the same time. Naturally occurring epidemics start from one central location and spread out in a circular fashion. They don't start

---

[226] Sharon Begley, "Are Tainted Vaccines Given to Baby Boomers Now Causing Cancer?" *Wall Street Journal*, 19 July 2002.

with heterosexual Africans, jump across the ocean, pass heterosexual and homosexual blacks, heterosexual whites, Hispanics, and every other group and then infect professional homosexual urban white men. Of course, even this scenario is impossible, because the AIDS epidemic erupted at the same time with American gays as it did in Africa. The most logical and probable explanation is that both groups were infected with contaminated vaccinations.

When one looks at all the "coincidences":

1.   The U.S. government and WHO funded research to create a virus that attacks the immune system in the same manner that AIDS attacks the immune system.

2.   U.S. government and WHO scientists conducted research about viruses that attack the immune system and published their findings. These papers were published before the AIDS epidemic.

3.   The first victims of the AIDS virus participated in vaccination programs administered by the WHO and the U.S. government.

The most logical theory on the origin of AIDS is that it is man-made bioweapon created by the U.S. government with the help of the WHO.

What is the black leadership's response to this epidemic? There is no call to investigate all the evidence that indicates that AIDS is a man-made bioweapon designed to target blacks. If they did that, they would no longer receive any of the white establishment's money. AIDS is just another opportunity for the black leadership to engage in irrational whining without ever touching the heart of the issue. They label AIDS a "civil rights" issue. Jesse Jackson has even said that AIDS has spread through black community because of "poverty, ignorance, and prejudice." What poverty and prejudice have to do with getting AIDS is beyond me. After the obligatory Marxist rhetoric, the black leadership calls for more education on the use of contraceptives and birth control, so called "safe sex." But never will you hear any member of the black establishment call for abstinence education. Studies have proven that abstinence education programs reduce sexual activity among teens, while sex education programs increase sexual activity.[227] Their solution to AIDS epidemic will only increase the incidences of AIDS in the black community.

The call for more use of condoms begs the question whether condoms even prevent the spread of AIDS. They don't according to former Surgeon General C. Everett Koop. Koop was a leading proponent of condoms and even went before Congress to urge the broadcast industry to lift a self-imposed ban on condom advertising. He stated before Congress that condoms could help slow the spread of AIDS even though it was admitted that condoms were not a failure-proof method. He did this knowing he would face a barrage of criticism because he was of member of the supposedly conservative Ronald Reagan administration. A few months after urging the broadcast industry to allow condoms ads, Koop suddenly reversed his position and decided to warn the American public on condom use. At a press conference at UCLA, Koop now stated that

---

[227] Sharon Kirkey, "Teaching Abstinence Reduces Teen Sex," *CanWest News Service*, 15 August 2006.

condoms have an "extraordinarily high" failure rate and stated that condoms "should not be seen as a panacea." He admitted that his earlier promotion of condom use was done before any major studies on their effectiveness. Koop stated: "I don't like to acknowledge mistakes, and I don't want to use the word 'mistake' in reference to that report. . . . But when I do it over, on the basis of information we have now and we (expect) to be getting, it will be much more explicit as to the expected failure rate in heterosexual (vaginal) and homosexual intercourse." [228]

Most people are unaware that the very same people who promoted the use of what once considered immoral—condoms—also don't believe condoms are safe. The media constantly promote the use of condoms, but they very rarely present the evidence that they don't protect people from AIDS. Since Koop advocated for condom manufacturers to be allowed to place ads, many studies have been conducted on their effectiveness. According to a July 20, 2001, study entitled "Scientific Evidence on Condom Effectiveness for Sexually

---

[228] Allan Parachini, "Koop Warns on Risk of AIDS in Condom Use," *Los Angeles Times*, 22 September 1987.

Transmitted Disease Prevention," conducted by the Department of Health of Human Services, condoms reduce the transmission rate of HIV by only 85 percent. For a fatal disease, this is not very effective. Pat Buchanan put it best when he observed that this is "roughly the odds one has of escaping unscathed when playing Russian roulette with a six-shooter with one chamber lethally loaded."[229] The study also found "no clinical proof" that condoms prevent the spread of chlamydia, syphilis, genital herpes, human papillomavirus, chancroid, or trichomoniasis.[230]

It is not just the government's studies that show condoms are not effective in stopping AIDS. Dr. Susan Weller, from the University of Texas Medical School, estimated a 31 percent failure rate of condoms for protecting against HIV.[231] According to Dr. Roland, editor of *Rubber Chemistry & Technology*, condoms have tiny microscopic holes in them five microns wide and the AIDS virus is only one micron wide.[232]

---

[229] Patrick J. Buchanan, "The Great Condom Fraud and Cover-Up," http://www.worldnetdaily.com/news/article.asp?ARTICLE_ID=26666, 1 March 2002.

[230] Cheryl Wetzstein, "CDC's leader Urged to Resign," *Washington Times*, 25 July 2001.

[231] Roger Richards, "Condoms: Safe or Sorry," *Business Korea* 14 (January 1997):

Condoms are not safe, the only "safe-sex" is abstinence until marriage. The Physicians Consortium, a group of 200 doctors, wrote a letter to President Bush demanding the resignation of CDC director Dr. Jeffrey Koplan for not launching a public relations campaign warning people that condoms are not safe after their own studies showed this to be the case. Planned Parenthood was even forced to admit that "abstinence from intercourse remains the most effective method" to avoid AIDS and other STDs.[233] Of course Planned Parenthood and the government still promote condom use on their Web sites and through their public relations programs.

So the there is a fatal disease ravaging the black community and the government promotes the use of condoms even though they know that condoms are not effective protection. What does the black leadership do? Do they launch initiatives to warn people not to listen to the pro-condom propaganda and that abstinence until marriage is the only way to ensure that you do not catch AIDS or another STD? No, they

---

[232] Ibid.
[233] Wetzstein, CDC's leader urged to resign," 4.

tell blacks to use condoms and practice "safe-sex." They give advice that may kill them.

The Catholic Church was attacked by the WHO, the same organization that conducted the vaccination programs that are linked to the spread of the AIDS virus in Africa, when they started telling people in countries hit hard by AIDS that condoms don't stop AIDS because they have tiny holes in them. Cardinal Alfonso Lopez Trujillo stated an undeniable fact that "the Aids virus is roughly 450 times smaller than the spermatozoon. The spermatozoon can easily pass through the 'net' that is formed by the condom . . . These margins of uncertainty . . . should represent an obligation on the part of the health ministries and all these campaigns to act in the same way as they do with regard to cigarettes, which they state to be a danger"[234]

The WHO response was to outright lie and deny a fact even admitted by Planned Parenthood and accuse the Church of

_____

[234] Steve Bradshaw, "Vatican: Condoms Don't Stop Aids," http://www.guardian.co.uk/print/0,,4770493-103681,00.html, 9 October 2003.

lying. "These incorrect statements about condoms and HIV are dangerous when we are facing a global pandemic which has already killed more than 20 million people, and currently affects at least 42 million."[235] Newspaper editorials routinely condemn the Catholic Church for their "superstitious" religious views on condom use. Those same newspapers never mention the multiple studies that have condoms to be poor protection against AIDS.

Chapter 9: The Final Solution and Gun Control

Abortion, sterilizations, and birth control are ways to get blacks to voluntary commit self-genocide. The eugenicists would prefer more direct methods of eliminating people, but the political climate rarely makes it feasible to implement those types of methods. In 1911 the Eugenics Section of the American Breeders Association, with Carnegie funding, devised an

---

[235] Ibid.

eighteen-point plan called, the "Preliminary Report of the Committee of the Eugenic Section of the American Breeders Association to Study and to Report on the Best Practical Means for Cutting Off the Defective Germ—Plasm—in the Human Population." The report called for a worldwide eugenics program. Point 8 of their plan explicitly called for euthanasia. But euthanasia was only a euphemism for murder as Edwin Black explains in his book *The War Against the Weak*, "Eugenicists did not see euthanasia as a 'merciful killing' of those in pain, but rather a 'painless killing' of people deemed unworthy of life."[236] The most talked-about method of killing people was the lethal gas chamber. Prominent socialist and darling of the left, George Bernard Shaw, said in a speech in 1910 that, "A part of eugenic politics would finally land us in an extensive use of the lethal chamber. A great many people would have to be put out of existence, simply because it wastes other people's time to look after them."[237] Modern-day eugenicists like Prince Philip, Duke of Edinburgh, husband of Queen

---

[236] Black, *War against the Weak*, 247.
[237] Ibid., 248.

Elizabeth, still hold on to this dream. Prince Phillip has stated

his desire to be reincarnated "to return as a deadly virus, in

order to contribute something to solve overpopulation."[238]

Make no mistake, if given the right opportunity, the

eugenicists would openly commit mass murder on the scale of

Hitler's holocaust to accomplish their objectives. Fortunately, in

America "extensive use of the lethal chamber" is not feasible

because of probable public backlash against such a program and

also because Americans benefit from a constitutional

guaranteed right to own a gun. Many Americans own guns and

it would be difficult, if not impossible, to carry out mass murder

on an armed population. It is for this reason that fighting gun

control legislation and the media campaign to demonize guns

and gun owners are of the utmost importance to anyone

opposed to eugenics.

The right of every man to bear arms has long been an

undisputed principle in Western thought. All the Founding

---

[238] Alex Jones, *9-11 Descent into Tyranny: The New World Order's Dark Plans to Turn Earth into a Prison Planet* Progressive Press, 2002.

Fathers believed in the importance of having an armed populace to preserve freedom. Today, revisionists claim that the Founding Fathers did not intend the Second Amendment to guarantee every man the right to be armed, but the words of the founding fathers clearly demonstrate they believed in the individual's right to bear arms just as much as they believed in his right to free speech and to practice his religion.

There have always been evil people who to seek to do good people harm. Any measures that disarm peaceful people would only leave them defenseless and would be an open invitation for criminals and tyrants to attack. Even Jesus advised his apostles to arm themselves: "And He said to them, 'But now, whoever has a money belt is to take it along, likewise also a bag, and whoever has no sword is to sell his coat and buy one.'"[239] Thomas Paine believed that if men were to give up their guns, "The peaceable part of mankind will be continually overrun by the vile and abandoned while they neglect the means of self-defense . . . [Weakness] allures the ruffian [but] arms like laws

---

[239] Luke 22:36

discourage and keep the invader and plunderer in awe and preserve order in the world. . . . Horrid mischief would ensue were [the good] deprived the use of them . . . [and] the weak will become a prey to the strong."[240] Thomas Jefferson noted that laws that forbid the carrying of arms "disarm those only who are neither inclined nor determined to commit crimes" and that they "make things worse for the assaulted and better for the assailants; they serve rather to encourage than to prevent homicides, for an unarmed man may be attacked with greater confidence than an armed man."[241] Patrick Henry made it clear what the purpose of the Second Amendment was, "The great object is that every man be armed."242 James Madison in the Federalist Papers No. 46 noted that great advantage Americans have over every other nation is that we are armed and that the oppressive governments of Europe "are afraid to trust the people with arms." George Mason believed that forbidding the carrying of arms is "the best and most effectual way to enslave"

---

[240] Wayne R. LaPierre, *Guns, Crime, and Freedom* HarperPerennial, 1995, 15–16.
[241] Ibid.
[242] Ibid., 16–17.

people.243 Even liberal Democratic vice president Hubert Humphrey wrote in 1960, "But the right of the citizen to bear arms is just one more safeguard against a tyranny which now appears remote in America, but historically has proved to be always possible."244 Not only were the founders unanimous in believing that every citizen had a right to bear arms, but that was the consensus belief held by both political parties until the late 1960s.

As much as freedom-loving men have always been in agreement about the importance of an armed populace, tyrants have been in agreement that it is necessary to disarm a populace in order to control, oppress, and/or kill them. Adolph Hitler wrote, "The most foolish mistake we could possibly make would be to allow the subject races to possess arms. History shows that all conquerors who have allowed their subject races to carry arms have prepared their own downfall by so doing."245 Chinese dictator, Mao Zedong, knew that "Political power

243 Wayne R. LaPierre, *Shooting Straight: Telling the Truth about Guns in America* Regnery Pub., 2002, 105.
244 Aaron Zelman and Richard W. Stevens, *Death by Gun Control* Mazel Freedom Press, 2001 28.
245 Zelman and Stevens, *Death by Gun Control*, 75.

flows out of the barrel of a gun, [but] our principle is that the Party commands the gun and the gun must never be allowed to command the Party."[246] When King George wanted to disarm the American colonists, English general Thomas Gage advised him, "Though the idea of disarming certain counties was a right one, yet it requires me to be a master of the country, in order to enable me to execute it."[247] General Gage knew that the American people could not be oppressed because they were armed.

If you want to oppress, enslave, or a kill a group of people, you must take away their guns. It is for this reason that the earliest gun control laws in America were explicitly applied only to blacks in order to prevent slave revolts. Slave owners in the south were always afraid of slave revolts, so they had strict restriction on gun ownership by slaves and free blacks. In Louisiana that it was lawful to beat "any black carrying any potential weapon, such as a cane."[248] In 1834 the Tennessee

---

[246] Ibid., 57.

[247] David Hardy, *Origins and Development of the Second Amendment* Blacksmith Corporation, 1986

[248] Clayton E. Cramer, "The Racist Roots of Gun Control," *Kansas Journal of Law and Public Policy* (Winter 1995),

Constitution was amended to only protect free white men's right to bear arms, previously the constitution guaranteed all free men, black or white, the right to bear arms.[249] Practically every state in the South had prohibitions against blacks owning firearms, a typical statue, like this 1840 law read, "That if any free negro, mulatto, or free person of color, shall wear or carry about his or her person, or keep in his or her house, any shot gun, musket, rifle, pistol, sword, dagger or bowie-knife, unless he or she shall have obtained a licence therefor from the Court of Pleas and Quarter Sessions of his or her county, within one year preceding the wearing, keeping or carrying therefor, he or she shall be guilty of a misdemeanor, and may be indicted therefor."[250]

These laws made sense from the slave owners' perspective because it is impossible to enslave an armed people.

It is not so much guns that the slave owners' feared, but the ability of slaves to defend themselves and their rights. In feudal

---

http://www.claytoncramer.com/scholarly/racistroots.htm.
[249] Ibid.
[250] Ibid.

Europe the aristocracy prohibited pheasants from owning swords because at that time the sword was the best means a man had to defend himself. The gun is one of the most effective weapons of self-defense, and that is why tyrants seek to ban and restrict ownership of guns. New Orleans made it illegal to teach free blacks fencing.[251] In Maryland, the authorities' fear of blacks was so great that free blacks were not even allowed to own a dog without a license.[252]

After the Civil War and the passing of the Fourteenth Amendment, legislatures could no longer make laws that explicitly forbid blacks from bearing arms. So laws were made with race neutral language that still accomplished the same objective as the previously overt racist laws. Laws were passed that banned selling of inexpensive firearms that the newly free, but mostly poor, blacks could afford. In 1870 Tennessee banned the selling of all guns but the expensive Army and Navy model handgun that most blacks could not afford. Most white veterans already had these guns, because they were given to veterans in

---

[251] Ibid.
[252] Ibid.

honor of their service.[253] South Carolina banned the sale of all handguns to everybody but "sheriffs and their special deputies."[254] Who were special deputies? They were any private citizens the sheriffs deputized, including members of the KKK. Alabama and Texas took another route by placing heavy taxes on guns, placing them out of the reach of both poor blacks and whites.[255] Mississippi and other Southern states simply ignored the Fourteenth Amendment and enforced explicitly racist gun control laws that forbid blacks from owning firearms.[256] Most of these laws were selectively enforced on blacks. When a white man was found with an illegal gun in his car in 1941, the Florida Supreme Court refused to apply the law and convict him. They made it clear in their decision that gun control laws, whether written in race neutral language or not, were meant to only apply to blacks:

---

[253] William R. Tonso, "Gun Control: White Man's Law," *REASON Magazine* (December 1985),
http://www.guncite.com/journals/gun_control_wtr8512.html.
[254] Ibid.
[255] Ibid.
[256] Stefan B. Tahmassebi, "Gun Control and Racism," *George Mason University Civil Rights Law Journal* 2 (1991),
http://www.saf.org/LawReviews/Tahmassebi1.html.

I know something of the history of this legislation. The original Act of 1893 was passed when there was a great influx of negro laborers in this State drawn here for the purpose of working in the turpentine and lumber camps. The same condition existed when the act was amended in 1901 and the act was passed for the purpose of disarming the negro laborers and to thereby reduce the unlawful homicides that were prevalent in turpentine and saw-mill camps and to give the white citizens in sparsely settled areas a better feeling of security. The statute was never intended to be applied to the white population and in practice has never been so applied.[257]

Today, no judge would be brave or foolish enough to be honest about the true purpose of gun control laws. Now he would pose as a liberal and defender of blacks and portray whites in favor of gun rights as racist rednecks. Racist gun control advocates still use some of the same tactics and have

---

[257] Robert J. Cottrol and Raymond T. Diamond, "The Second Amendment: Toward an Afro-Americanist Reconsideration," *Georgetown Law Journal* (December 1991).

banned cheap handguns called "Saturday Night Specials." The name "Saturday Night Specials" is derived for the derogatory term "Niggertown Saturday Night" used to describe weekend violence in poor black neighborhoods.

After the race riots of late 1960s, fear spread throughout the halls of Congress. Senator Thomas Dodd took advantage of this fear to introduce radical gun control legislation. Governments often take advantage of a crisis to pass laws to take away people's freedoms. After a crisis, whether a riot or a terrorist attack, people are fearful and are often willing to give up their freedoms for government protection. According to publicly available documents, Dodd asked the Library Congress for an English translation of the notorious "Law of Weapons of March 18, 1938," used by the Nazis to disarm the Jews and other enemies of the Nazi regime.[258] Dodd was familiar with the law and the crimes of the Nazis because he worked with the prosecuting attorneys at the Nuremberg trials. Congress then passed the Gun Control Act of 1968, the text of which is eerily

---

[258] Zelman and Stevens. *Death by Gun* Control

similar to the text of the 1938 Nazi law. Left-wing antigun journalist Robert Sherrill admitted that the Gun Control Act of 1968 was "passed not to control guns but to control Blacks."[259] Roy Innis of the Congress of Racial Equality (CORE) was one of the few blacks to object to the bill, stating, "Black people would be disarmed and white people would not be."[260]

In addition to banning the sale of inexpensive guns, many communities passed laws that required one to get a permit before purchasing a gun. Gun permits are issued by the police, entirely at their discretion. A typical law, the New York law, says that police "shall issue" a permit if the applicant has "good moral character" and has "proper cause" to request a permit. How do you determine whether an applicant has good moral character? It is completely at police discretion. It should surprise no one, that typically only the rich and well-connected get permits. Almost all of the 8,000 permits issued in New York City are to residents of the wealthy Upper West Side.[261] The

[259] Tahmassebi, "Gun Control and Racism."
[260] "Johnson's Gun Control Plan Opposed by CORE Official," *New York Times*, 15 July 1968.
[261] Michael L. Betsch, "Blacks Allegedly Victimized by 'Racist' Gun Control Laws,"

California state legislature admits that the majority of permits are issued to whites.[262] Gun control opponent John Lott explains that "when you have these discretionary states, blacks get permits at much lower rates than they get them in the states which are the 'right to carry' states which don't allow discretion on the part of public officials. You try to get a permit and you live in Harlem, it's like no chance. You'd think these people are going to have the biggest benefit from having it, but when you have this type of [political] discretion in terms of whether or not they'll let somebody get it, they just will refuse." [263] In St. Louis a personal interview is required before a gun permit is issued. One person reported the personal interview only consisted of the sheriff looking at him to see he wasn't black, then yelling, "he's all right."[264]

Many, if not most, gun control advocates probably actually believe the antigun rhetoric and don't own guns. The elites, on the other hand, the biggest propagandists in favor of gun control

http://www.cnsnews.com/public/Content/Article.aspx?rsrcid=5413&print=on&print=on, 30 January 2003.
[262] Cramer, "The Racist Roots of Gun Control."
[263] Betsch, "Blacks Allegedly Victimized."
[264] Tahmassebi, "Gun Control and Racism."

and prohibition, often own guns. When she was a mayor of San Francisco, Dianne Feinstein signed a bill that banned most residents from owning handguns. Yet she kept her gun and was one of only eight people in the city allowed to own a gun. The *New York Times* often editorializes in favor of gun control, but owner Arthur Sulzberger has a gun permit. Antigun politicians Nelson Rockefeller and John Lindsey also had permits. If you are taxi cab driver in New York City, one of the most dangerous jobs in the world, you can forget about getting a permit. Police won't give it to you because you carry less than $2,000.[265] In New York City some people have the right to defend their lives and property and some don't.

Since the black population is concentrated in big cities that tend to be liberal, it is possible that fewer blacks than ever in our history have full gun rights. In fact, most educated blacks have been so domesticated that they snicker at the phrase "gun rights" and see no problem that for most blacks who live in big

---

[265] Jeffrey R. Snyder, "Fighting Back: Crime, Self-Defense, and the Right to Carry a Handgun," Cato Policy Analysis http://www.cato.org/pub_display.php?pub_id=1143, 22 October 1997.

cities have no right to bear arms. These educated blacks, many of them, if not most, are physical cowards who are not concerned with freedom but they mostly want more handouts and entitlements. They cannot understand why anyone would want a gun. Their ancestors who faced the Ku Klux Klan and violent race riots can answer that question better than anyone.

Between 1882 and 1968, the KKK and angry white mobs lynched 4,743 people, and the vast majority of the victims were black. Many of their victims were unarmed and the police participated in the attacks, or stood by and did nothing while the lynchings took place. South Carolina's governor, Coleman L. Blease, bragged that he refused to call out the state militia to protect blacks.[266] In the North, violent race riots between whites and blacks were a frequent occurrence. In August of 1843, in Boston, mobs of whites attacked every black man they could find. In 1834, in New York, white mobs went on a rampage, destroying the churches, homes, and businesses of white abolitionists and blacks. During the Hardscrabble Riot of

---

[266] Zelman and Stevens, *Death by Gun Control*, 206.

October of 1824, mobs of whites destroyed every house in the predominately black Providence, Rhode Island, neighborhood.[267]

During Reconstruction, northern Republicans were fully aware that because blacks in the South were prohibited from owning guns and consequently unable to defend themselves that many injustices were allowed to take place. Reconstruction marks the only time in American history that the white or black establishment showed any interest in the gun rights of blacks. Massachusetts congressman Benjamin F. Butler tried unsuccessfully to pass a law that would make it a felony to take away a gun from a black man because he observed, "in many counties they have preceded their outrages upon him by disarming him, in violation of his right as a citizen to 'keep and bear arms' which the Constitution expressly says shall never be infringed."[268] Senator John Sherman of Ohio agreed with Butler and said, "Wherever the Negro population preponderates, there they [the KKK] hold their sway, for a few determined men . . .

---

[267] Cottrol and Diamond, "The Second Amendment,"[AQ: page number(s)?].
[268] Robert J. Cottrol, *Gun control and the Constitution : Sources and Explorations on the Second Amendment:* Garland Pub., 1994), 365.

can carry terror among ignorant Negroes . . . without arms, equipment, or discipline."[269] Senator Henry Wilson from Massachusetts noted that "in Mississippi rebel State forces, men who were in the rebel armies, are traversing the State, visiting the freedmen, disarming them, perpetrating murders and outrages upon them."[270] New York congressman Henry J. Raymond explained clearly what rights the newly freed slaves had. "He has a defined status: he has a country and a home; a right to defend himself and his wife and children; a right to bear arms."[271] Despite some valiant efforts by northern politicians to protect black's right to bear arms, they were ultimately unsuccessful. The 1875 Cruikshank decision by the Supreme Court settled the question by stating that the states had the right to take away guns from blacks.

When and where blacks had the opportunity to arm themselves they did not just sit idly by and wait for someone to protect them; they formed militias to defend themselves, their

---

[269] Ibid.
[270] Tahmassebi, "Gun Control and Racism."
[271] Ibid.

families, and their neighbors. Today, the media attaches negative connotations to militias. We are told that only white racists form militias and believe in the right to carry arms. But the truth is militias are formed by brave self-reliant men who know that there are evil people in the world who seek to do others harm. They know that the government is not always there to protect you, and in some cases the government is looking to do you harm. The black men who formed militias would not recognize the typical black man of today who waits for the government to solve his problems. There are countless examples of blacks exercising their right to bear arms and defending themselves against attackers. During the Providence, Rhode Island, Snowtown Riot of 1831, a white mob destroyed seventeen houses occupied by blacks and did not stop until blacks fired into the crowd.[272] In Cincinnati, in 1841, whites burned and looted black-owned businesses for two nights straight. When the mob tried to enter the black residential district, they were beaten back by blacks who fired at the mob.

---

[272] Cottrol and Diamond, "The Second Amendment,".

The next day the government disarmed the blacks and the white mob returned to wreak havoc on the now-defenseless black community.[273] In Columbia, South Carolina, the jailer's fourteen-year-old daughter, using only a revolver, held back a white mob that wanted to lynch a black prisoner.[274] A black militia unit in Memphis, in 1891, protected 100 black prisoners who were in danger of being lynched for several nights.[275] Dr. Ossian Sweet, of Detroit, shot and killed a member of angry white mob that was attacking his home as the police stood by and did nothing. Michigan later passed a handgun permit law in response to this incident.[276] When Ida B. Wells-Barnett was warned that she was in danger because of her antilynching protest activities, she started to carry a pistol. Ida B. Wells-Barnett explained her decision. "I had been warned repeatedly by my own people that something would happen if I did not cease harping on the lynching of three months before. . . . I had

---

[273] Ibid.

[274] Zelman and Stevens, *Death by Gun* Control, 207.

[275] Ibid., 208.

[276] David Kopel, "Selective Disarmament: No Guns for the Poor," http://www.nraila.org/Issues/Articles/Read.aspx?id=16&issue=020, 6 October 1999.

bought a pistol the first thing after [the lynching], because I expected some cowardly retaliation from the lynchers. I felt that one had better die fighting against injustice than to die like a dog or a rat in a trap. I had already determined to defend my life as dearly as possible if attacked. I felt if I could take one lyncher with me, this would even up the score a little bit."[277]

This brave lady was more of a man than the typical black male "leader" today. A black newspaper reported during racist riots in New York City that "colored men who had the manhood in them armed themselves, and threw out their pickets every day and night, determined to die in their homes."[278] This is obviously a different attitude than the whiny effeminate nature of today's typical black leader, who would most likely sit back and watch innocent people die, while complaining about racism and demanding something be done without doing anything himself. This manly courageous attitude was even present as late as the 1960s. Civil rights lawyer Don B. Kates noted, "As a civil rights worker in a Southern state during the early 1960's, I

---

[277] Cottrol and Diamond, "The Second Amendment,".
[278] Cottrol, *Gun Control and the Constitution*, 361.

179

found that the possession of firearms for self-defense was almost universally endorsed by the black community, for it could not depend on police protection from the KKK . . . . The black lawyer for whom I principally worked . . . attributed the relative quiescence of the Klan to the fact that the black community was so heavily armed."[279]

The Deacons for Defense and Justice, a militia formed in Louisiana in 1964, had fifty to sixty chapters throughout Louisiana, Mississippi, and Alabama. They protected blacks and civil rights workers against the KKK and weren't afraid to fight back.[280] Civil rights activist John Salter, who defended his home and family from the KKK with his gun in the 1960s, wrote, "No one knows what kind of massive racist retaliation would have been directed against grass-roots black people had the black community not had a healthy measure of firearms within it."[281]

---

[279] Tahmassebi, "Gun Control and Racism."
[280] Cottrol and Diamond, "The Second Amendment,"[AQ: page number(s)].
[281] Kopel."Selective Disarmament."

Although John Salter is right, no one can know for certain what kind of atrocities would have taken place if blacks were completely disarmed. We can only speculate, but if countries with no gun rights and hated minority populations are any guide, it is possible there could have been mass murder in America that would have made the lynchings done by the KKK look like a pleasure cruise. Aaron Zelman and Richard W. Stevens in their book *Death by Gun Control* document the many instances of genocide of hated groups in the twentieth century, all of them preceded by gun confiscation and gun control measures, and below is a summary of a few examples of genocides in the last century:

Cambodia: Cambodia had strict gun control laws that made it nearly impossible for the common man to own a gun; consequently gun ownership rates were low among Cambodians. Cambodians have always lived under tyrannical governments but nothing compared to the homicidal regime of the Khmer Rouge and their leader Pol Pot. Pol Pot outlawed religion, free speech, travel, and even money. Pol Pot collectivized farms and anyone over five years old was enslaved and forced to work on farms from early morning to nightfall. Famine and abject poverty followed the Khmer Rouge's communist policies. Pol Pot would execute whole towns of people if they rebelled against his rule. All educated and "rich" people were tortured to death and executed. Pol Pot's definition of rich included anyone who spoke French or English, anyone who wore glasses, and college students. At the labor camps, laughing, crying, and displaying sadness over the death of your child was punishable by death. Between 40,000 and 60,000 Buddhist monks were executed, and one half of the Muslim population was killed. Between 1970 and 1980, 29 percent of the population, or 2 million people, were killed.[282]

China: The Chinese have never known freedom and have always lived under authoritarian oppressive governments, but when the Communists took over that country the people saw a

---

[282] Zelman and Stevens, *Death by Gun Control*, 33–44.

tyranny that even they could not fathom. The Chinese people

were prohibiting from owning guns. Again, like Cambodia, the

Chinese Communists instituted forced collectivized farming,

and it doesn't take Adam Smith to predict the mass starvation

that took place. Between 1949 and 1987 more than 35 million

people died either by starvation or execution or were worked to

their death.[283]

Nazi Germany: The atrocities done to the Jews during World

War II are well known and told to Americans through the media

and the schools on what seems like a daily basis. But what isn't

told are the gun control laws and gun confiscation that preceded

the Holocaust. First the gypsies were disarmed in 1928. The

Nazis burned the Reichstag in 1933 and blamed it on

Communist terrorists and used the event to disarm the

Communists. During the same year, a law was passed that

required all non-Nazi Germans to turn in "military" weapons

but allowed them to keep civilian weapons. Bolt-action rifles

---

[283] Ibid., 47–55.

and revolvers fell under the definition of "military" weapons. Shortly after this law was passed, the Nazis raided Jewish homes and neighborhoods searching for "military" weapons. Finally in 1938, a comprehensive gun control law was passed that required a license to buy, sell, or manufacture firearms. Although the law did not name Jews specifically, it effectively made it impossible for Jews to acquire guns. The police were given discretion in granting permits and could deny a permit to anyone "whose reliability is not in doubt, and only after proving a need for them," this usually made it impossible for Jews to get permits. On November 7, 1938, a Jew assassinated a German official. The Nazis capitalized on the fear and anger caused by this event, by issuing a decree, explicitly banning all Jews from owning all firearms and then launched a final raid on the Jewish community. They seized all weapons, including "stabbing and cutting weapons," regardless if they had a permit or not. The disarming of the Jewish population allowed the Holocaust to take place. [284]

---

[284] Ibid., 75–111.

Rwanda: Rwanda is composed of two major tribes: the Hutus, which make up 90 percent of the population, and the minority Tutsis, which are about 9 percent of the population. Between April and July of 1994 the Hutu-controlled government launched a campaign of genocide against the Tutsis and killed 80 percent of them. All Rwandans were required to carry ethnic identity cards. Death squads went around checking peoples' identity cards, and if they were Tutsis, they were taken away and executed. Because Rwanda prohibited civilians from owning guns, the Tutsis were forced to defend themselves with bows and arrows and stones against men armed with guns. Guess who won those battles? Even the UN had to admit, "most of the massacres were carried out . . . against unarmed and defenseless people." What was the United Nations doing there? They were there on a peacekeeping mission, obstinately to keep peace between Hutus and Tutsis. When the genocide began they didn't lift one finger to help the Tutsis. [285] The UN's behavior

---

[285] Ibid., 123–32.

shows that people usually will not put themselves in danger to defend anyone but themselves. They may defend members of their family or members of a group they identify with, like a neighborhood, religion, tribe, or nationality. But, it is extremely unlikely for anyone to put themselves in danger to defend strangers. You must be self-reliant and ready, able, and willing to defend yourself.

Turkey: The Turks had always resented the Armenian Christian minority, and in 1915 they decided to do something about it. They devised a plan to send all Armenian young men into war and put them on the front lines against the Russians. Some men avoided service, so the Turks arrested all the Armenian men they could find and demanded every Armenian turn in all their guns. Armenians were given a quota of guns to turn in and those who did not turn in that amount were tortured and imprisoned. Now the leaders of this Muslim country were free to exterminate the defenseless Armenian children, women, and elderly. Armenian soldiers were disarmed and either worked to death or executed. When it was all over, between 1 and 1.5 million people died in two years.[286]

Soviet Union: The Communists can't produce enough food to feed a nation; they can't even make enough toilet paper. But one thing, the only thing, they are good at, is killing their own countrymen. Russia is just another example where they displayed their prowess in mass murder. On October 29, 1918, Fanny Kaplan tried to assassinate Lenin. Unfortunately, Lenin survived. The Communists used this event to justify a decree demanding all firearms be turned over to the Communist government. Government officials were rewarded for collecting guns and punished if the Communists did not think they did a good enough job. Because the Russians did not own guns Stalin, was able to kill 10 million people between 1934 and 1941.[287]

---

[286] Ibid., 133–47.
[287] Ibid., 159–79.

Above are examples of the travesties that can take place when a population is disarmed. As blacks did in America foreign that are targeted victims of genocide have shown that when they can get their hands on guns, they are able and willing to fight back and sometimes survive, but if they don't survive at least they die fighting. In the Warsaw Ghetto in Poland, the Jews formed a militia called the Jewish Fighting Organization (ZOB) and decided to fight the Germans. They were able to retrieve guns and grenades from the bodies of dead soldiers. Even though the Jews were outnumbered ten to one, they held back the Germans, one of the greatest armies ever assembled, for twenty-nine days before being defeated. Some members of the ZOB chose to fight to the death rather than surrender. In Uganda homicidal dictator Idi Amin killed 30,000 of his political enemies. But when his troops went to the home of Ricarda Hetsch, she fired three shots and Idi Amin's troops ran away. Like most bullies, Idi Amin's troops were nothing but cowards and quickly backed down when someone stood up to them.[288] In Zimbabwe, racist dictator Robert Mugabe seized the land of white farmers. He encouraged bands of racist black thugs to invade white-owned farms and squat on the land. The squatters would demand that the farmers leave and would use violence, often beating up the farmers and their employees. Since Mugabe is a complete idiot, he didn't take away the farmers' guns before he encouraged the squatters. Some farmers decided to fight back. Martin Olds was not giving up his farm without a fight. When seventy armed men came to his farm, he fought them armed only with his shotgun. He fought until he ran out of ammunition and was killed. He didn't even let a gunshot wound in his leg stop him. After his display of courage, the police went around disarming all existing farmers of their weapons.

Chapter 10: Conclusion

"All that is necessary for the triumph of evil is that good men do nothing"

Attributed to Edmund Burke

---

[288] Ibid., 149–58.

"The wisest thing in the world is to cry out before you are hurt. It is no good to cry out after you are hurt; especially after you are mortally hurt. People talk about the impatience of the populace; but sound historians know that most tyrannies have been possible because men moved too late. It is often essential to resist a tyranny before it exists. It is no answer to say, with a distant optimism, that the scheme is only in the air. A blow from a hatchet can only be parried while it is in the air."

G. K. Chesterton—*Eugenics and Other Evils*

The most common reaction by people when they learn of the eugenicists' murderous plans is to dismiss and shrug it off by saying, "They will never be successful" or "It could never happen here." This is just a way of sticking your head in the sand and hoping all your problems will go away. This is a common human reaction. How many times have you had a friend who suffered from an ailment, perhaps a rash, but was hesitant to go to the doctor because he feared that the doctor would tell him that there was something horribly wrong with him? We all know that this is irrational and self-destructive behavior, but still many of us choose to live in denial and not face our problems.

The eugenicists are counting on people to live in denial. One of the advantages the eugenicists have is that their goals are so evil that most people have difficulty relating to and comprehending the eugenicists. Although we don't approve of a bank robber, we can understand why he does it. He wants money, and he doesn't want to work for it. The average person cannot understand why someone would want to kill off most of the human race. The eugenicists are probably so open about their objectives and methods because they knew most people will just ignore them or refuse to believe they could be that evil.

The eugenicists are not the only people who publically expressed their evil intentions and methods before they carried out their plans. Adolph Hitler told the whole world of his plans in his autobiography *Mien Kampf* in 1925, eight years before he became chancellor in 1933. He proceeded to carry out his plans exactly how he laid them out in *Mien Kampf*. The Communists published many books explaining what they would do when they took power. Hitler and the Communists could have been stopped if the world paid attention to their own words and took them seriously. We can also stop the eugenicists. We must expose them and inform as many people as possible.

While many will live in denial others will accept the reality of the eugenicists' plan but will say they are too powerful to defeat, so therefore it is no use to fight them. No group or conspiracy is so powerful that it can't be defeated. At its height, the British Empire controlled one quarter of the world's territory. The empire has fallen, and the United Kingdom is no longer a superpower. Totalitarian and all-powerful Communist governments like Russia have also fallen. Our Founding Fathers went up against one of the world's greatest superpowers and they were victorious. We have a duty to fight the eugenicists, and with the grace of God, we can defeat them.

www.ingramcontent.com/pod-product-compliance
Lightning Source LLC
Chambersburg PA
CBHW050119280326
41933CB00010B/1160